# HEALTH SCIENCES LITERATURE REVIEW MADE EASY

THE MATRIX METHOD

## JUDITH GARRARD, PhD

*Senior Associate Dean for Academic Affairs and Research*
*Professor, Division of Health Policy and Management*
*School of Public Health*
*University of Minnesota*
*Minneapolis, Minnesota*

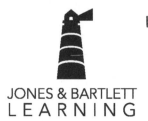

JONES & BARTLETT
LEARNING

*World Headquarters*

| Jones & Bartlett Learning | Jones & Bartlett Learning | Jones & Bartlett Learning |
|---|---|---|
| 40 Tall Pine Drive | Canada | International |
| Sudbury, MA 01776 | 6339 Ormindale Way | Barb House, Barb Mews |
| 978-443-5000 | Mississauga, Ontario | London W6 7PA |
| info@jblearning.com | L5V 1J2 | United Kingdom |
| www.jblearning.com | Canada | |

Jones & Bartlett Learning books and products are available through most bookstores and online booksellers. To contact Jones & Bartlett Learning directly, call 800-832-0034, fax 978-443-8000, or visit our website, www.jblearning.com.

Substantial discounts on bulk quantities of Jones & Bartlett Learning publications are available to corporations, professional associations, and other qualified organizations. For details and specific discount information, contact the special sales department at Jones & Bartlett Learning via the above contact information or send an email to specialsales@jblearning.com.

The author, editor, and publisher have made every effort to provide accurate information. However, they are not responsible for errors, omissions, or for any outcomes related to the use of the contents of this book and take no responsibility for the use of the products and procedures described. Treatments and side effects described in this book may not be applicable to all people; likewise, some people may require a dose or experience a side effect that is not described herein. Drugs and medical devices are discussed that may have limited availability controlled by the Food and Drug Administration (FDA) for use only in a research study or clinical trial. Research, clinical practice, and government regulations often change the accepted standard in this field. When consideration is being given to use of any drug in the clinical setting, the health care provider or reader is responsible for determining FDA status of the drug, reading the package insert, and reviewing prescribing information for the most up-to-date recommendations on dose, precautions, and contraindications, and determining the appropriate usage for the product. This is especially important in the case of drugs that are new or seldom used.

**Production Credits**

Publisher: Kevin Sullivan
Acquisitions Editor: Amy Sibley
Associate Editor: Patricia Donnelly
Editorial Assistant: Rachel Shuster
Associate Production Editor: Katie Spiegel
Marketing Manager: Rebecca Wasley

V.P., Manufacturing and Inventory Control: Therese Connell
Composition: Auburn Associates, Inc.
Cover Design: Scott Moden
Printing and Binding: Malloy, Inc.
Cover Printing: Malloy, Inc.

**Library of Congress Cataloging-in-Publication Data**
Garrard, Judith.
  Health sciences literature review made easy : the matrix method / Judith Garrard. — 3rd ed.
     p. ; cm.
  Includes bibliographical references and index.
  ISBN 978-0-7637-7186-7
  1. Medical literature—Research—Methodology. 2. Matrix method (Indexing) 3. Medicine—Abstracting and indexing. 4. Information storage and retrieval systems—Medicine. I. Title.
  [DNLM: 1. Review Literature as Topic. 2. Writing. 3. Abstracting and Indexing as Topic.
4. Information Storage and Retrieval. WZ 345 G238h 2011]
  R118.6.G37 2011
  610.72—dc22
                                    2009054076

6048
Printed in the United States of America
14  13  12  11  10     10 9 8 7 6 5 4 3 2 1

# Dedication

• • •

*This book is dedicated to my husband, Bill, our adult children, Zandy and Libby, our children-in-law, Heidi and Lee, our grandsons, Hayden, Liam, and Henry Glascoe, and our canine companions, Molly and Scooter.*

• • •

# Table of Contents

Part

I

Chapter

1

Chapter

2

# Preface

The third edition has undergone considerable revision, including the following:

- *Electronic Basis.* The method has been converted from a hard copy method (using a three-ring notebooks and paper-based spreadsheets) to an entirely electronic basis (including computer folders and sub-folders). There is a new appendix that serves as a guide for how to set up such files, and information is interwoven throughout all of the chapters that describe this move to an electronic basis.
- *Changes at the National Level.* This edition of this book describes the rapidly changing innovations in the National Library of Medicine infrastructure and the impact of these changes on how to review the literature in the health sciences.
- *Changes in the Field.* Different terms have been introduced to describe a review of the literature. These terms and how they compare to the kind of literature review described in this book are described.

The purpose, scope, and emphasis of the book have not changed in this edition. They remain as follows:

- *Purpose.* The purpose of this book is to describe a practical and useful method for reviewing the literature, especially the scientific literature in the health sciences. The audience continues to be the graduate or professional student who needs a practical, step-by-step set of instructions about how to conduct a review of the literature. That is its fundamental goal.
- *Scope.* The scope of this book spans the beginning student to the health professional in the workplace. The methods for conducting a review of the literature apply to all of the major health professions, including public health, nursing, dentistry, medicine, pharmacy, veterinary medicine, and the allied health sciences.
- *Emphasis.* The emphasis in this book is on practical applications. Our goal was and continues to be a method for actually conducting a review of the literature and preparing a synthesis.

# Acknowledgments

In the 11 years since the first edition of this book went to press and now in 2010 as the third edition goes to press, there have been many changes in the tools researchers use to develop a literature review and how those tools are typically used. Some of the most dramatic changes have been in the resources available in university-based biomedical libraries.

I had the good fortune to work with three dynamic biomedical librarians at the University of Minnesota Health Sciences Libraries in the preparation of these materials, and I want to gratefully acknowledge them: Chad Fennel, Lisa McGuire, and Del Reed. Chad is a 2004 MLIS graduate from the University of Illinois at Urbana-Champaign; Lisa received her MLIS from Dominican University in River Forest, Illinois in 1999, and Del completed a PhD in philosophy at the University of Minnesota in 2000. During the months that we met, they taught me a lot about the present and future resources in today's health sciences libraries, and I want to urge the readers of this book to seek out their own equivalent of this dynamic group of librarians at their own libraries.

The second and third editions would not have been possible without a first edition, and I am continually grateful for the help from another librarian, Julie Kelly, at the University of Minnesota's Magrath Library. The improvements and additions to the second edition reflect input from all of these people; the errors are mine alone.

I also want to acknowledge the continued support and encouragement of my husband, Bill Garrard, in this endeavor, as well as that of our children and grandchildren (and our canine companions).

My editors and their colleagues at Jones and Bartlett Publishers have been patient and encouraging throughout the process of the third edition. I am grateful for the help and encouragement of the editorial team at Jones and Bartlett Publishers, especially Rachel Shuster, Katie Spiegel, and Kevin Sullivan. I also want to express my appreciation to the anonymous (to me) reviewers recruited by my publisher to advise me on how the book could be improved. Many of their suggestions have been included in this edition.

Part

# I

# Fundamentals of a Literature Review

# 1

# Introduction

The Matrix Method is a versatile strategy for reviewing the literature. The background and philosophy of a literature review and an introduction to the Matrix Method are described in the following sections in this chapter:

- ⊙ Review of the Literature
- ⊙ Well Beyond Index Cards
- ⊙ To Own the Literature
- ⊙ Research Synthesis: Historical Perspective
- ⊙ The Matrix Method: Definition and Overview
- ⊙ Review Matrix: A Versatile Tool
- ⊙ Overview of Chapters and Appendices
- ⊙ References to Websites
- ⊙ Caroline's Quest: Understanding the Process

# REVIEW OF THE LITERATURE

The purpose of this book is to describe the Matrix Method and the Matrix Indexing System. The Matrix Method is a strategy for reviewing the literature, especially the scientific literature. A review of the literature consists of reading, analyzing, and writing a synthesis of scholarly materials about a specific topic. When the review is of scientific literature, the focus is on the hypotheses, scientific methods, results, strengths, and weaknesses of the study, and the authors' interpretations and conclusions. A review of the scientific literature is fundamental to understanding the accumulated knowledge about the topic being reviewed. The Matrix Indexing System helps the user to create and maintain a reprint file.

The term *scientific literature* refers to theoretical and research publications in scientific journals, reference books, textbooks, government reports, policy statements, and other materials about the theory, practice, and results of scientific inquiry. These materials and publications are produced by individuals or groups in universities, foundations, government research laboratories, and other nonprofit or for-profit organizations. Throughout this book, the term *source document* will be used to refer to any of these sources, such as a journal article, a chapter in a book, or a research report. Currently, the most common type of publication used in a review of up-to-date scientific literature is a research paper in a scientific journal, such as the *Journal of the American Medical Association* (*JAMA*) or the *American Journal of Epidemiology*.

Reviews of the literature are the foundation for theses and dissertations, grant proposals, research papers, summary articles, books, policy and regulatory statements, evidence-based healthcare statements for health professionals, and consumer materials. Given the vast number of scientific publications produced over the past several decades, information retrieval and analysis in the form of a critical review of the literature have become more crucial than ever.

Over the past 20–30 years, the following terms have been used interchangeably: *literature review, integrative review, systematic review,* and *meta-analysis.* All share the same basic elements, which are: (1) stating the purpose of the review; (2) screening and selecting scientific papers that meet specified criteria; (3) carefully reviewing the papers for excellence of scientific methods, statistical procedures, and validity and reliability of data collection; (4) summarizing findings across the studies; and (5) drawing conclusions based on the scientific evidence.

In this book, a *literature review* is defined as an analysis of scientific materials about a specific topic that requires the reviewer to carefully read each of the studies to evaluate the study purpose, determine the appropriateness and quality of the scientific methods, examine the analysis of the questions and answers posed by the authors, summarize the findings across the studies, and write an objective synthesis of the findings.

In describing an *integrative review*, authors emphasize the review of past research in which the goal of the review is to base conclusions on many different studies.[1] An *integrative review* (or *integrative literature review*) is a term that tends to be found in the nursing literature.

The term *systematic review* appears more frequently in publications about evidence-based medicine. The term has been defined as an overview of scientific evidence in the medical literature that emphasizes treatment, causation, diagnosis, and prognosis.[2] According to this definition, systematic reviews are prepared specifically for clinicians and provide the basis for the practice of evidence-based medicine. Other clinical fields have adopted the strategy of basing their clinical practices and decision-making processes on the evidence in the scientific literature.

A *meta-analysis* is a departure from the other three types of reviews because this kind of summary of the literature requires precise quantitative methods to summarize the results. The same standards for rigor in identifying the purpose of the review, careful selection of papers, and evaluation of methods is essential to this type of review.

In general, think about the first three of these types of review as being similar, with the names being used in specific fields or disciplines to basically refer to a very rigorous literature review. The meta-analysis is described more fully later in this book.

## WELL BEYOND INDEX CARDS

In the past, most students conducted their first review of the literature in high school or college when they learned how to do library research. Usually their efforts concentrated on where to gather information and how to use the library. With the advent of computers, students now learn about electronic information retrieval at the primary school level.

Using computers to retrieve information is not the only new development, however. The sheer amount of information to be examined and critiqued has increased exponentially over the past 50 years. The first decade of the 21st century alone has witnessed tremendous advancements in scientific knowledge, a dramatic increase in the number of scientific journals, and a bewildering array of new forms of communication. Books and scientific journals are no longer the only venue for scholarly literature. Information is available on the Internet, in national and international meetings of professional societies, and in correspondence by e-mail, on blogs, and through social networking software such as Twitter, Facebook, and wikis. The issue of how, where, when, and whether or not to obtain information from these sources constitutes a present-day dilemma for anyone who reviews the scientific literature. The art of conducting such a review is an entirely separate matter.

Formal instruction in how to organize systematically and carry out a review of the literature is rarely offered in educational programs at any level, including graduate school. In the past, American students were advised to use index cards to record the most salient points of the material being reviewed. Now students keep notes on a computer or on other electronic devices. Despite such technological advances, how to avoid getting lost in the details between generating a computer list of research articles, accumulating electronic notes, and writing the final synthesis is still something of a mystery to many people.

One way of mastering this process is to realize that a review of any body of literature actually consists of four fundamental tasks, once the subject of the review has been decided:

1. Make decisions about which documents to review
2. Read and understand what the authors describe in those documents
3. Evaluate the ideas, research methods, and results of each publication
4. Write a synthesis that includes both the content and a critical analysis of these materials

Given the complexity of each one of these tasks, it is easy to become overwhelmed in the process. A strategy is needed to organize the books and papers selected in the search and retrieval process, structure the information in order to understand the progression of ideas by different authors across documents and over time, and use that structure to develop a critique and write a synthesis of the results of such a review. The Matrix Method provides such a strategy.

## TO OWN THE LITERATURE

Something else can result from a thorough and comprehensive review of the literature that may be even more valuable than a written synthesis—ownership of the literature. To "own the literature," you must know it—know the major ideas, what has been researched, the names of the authors and their professional affiliations, who collaborated with whom, what databases they did (or did not) use, the methodological strengths and weaknesses of the studies, what has been studied ad infinitum, and especially what is missing.

To own the literature is to be so familiar with what has been written by previous researchers that you know clearly how this area of research has progressed over time and across ideas. Without a thorough and comprehensive review of the literature, you are at the mercy of every critic and reviewer who is aware of what is known, how it evolved, and what has yet to be examined.

Unfortunately, such ownership cannot be acquired easily; you have to complete the entire process of a literature review, from the initial search to the final written synthesis, before you can take possession of the literature on a subject. Ownership is rarely mentioned when people describe the literature in a paper or presentation, but it exists; experienced reviewers achieve such ownership whether or not they realize it.

When you own the literature, you are in a better position to know what is missing in a stream of research. You can defend your ideas and anticipate what other scientists and researchers will say or do. Ownership is the mastery of how a specific body of knowledge evolved, what it currently comprises, and what has yet to be studied.

Acquiring ownership of literature demands more than summarizing the studies or documents you reviewed. A summary merely describes. Your task is to read and analyze each document until you can picture what the authors did in a study or the logical process they went through in making a point. Then you must go back and critically analyze what was right and wrong each step of the way. To own the literature is to dissect each part and decide whether you agree with what the authors did or said. In other words, you must become engaged with the content, argue with the authors' logic, and conclude for yourself whether that paper or study made sense from a scientific or scholarly standpoint. You must understand how the field has evolved, including the progression of ideas over time and across different authors. To own the literature you must learn about the conceptual models that served as the foundation for the research, and you must deduce what hypotheses were really being tested, who initiated the ideas, and who did the first research study. The Matrix Method will help you acquire ownership of the literature, but it is only a guide. The most important component is your active involvement with the literature.

# RESEARCH SYNTHESIS: HISTORICAL PERSPECTIVE

## Overview

Before delving into the details of the Matrix Method, it might be useful to think about the historical context of a review of the literature. A literature review is part of the larger endeavor of research synthesis that is the analysis, interpretation, and use of scientific inquiry. Although the term *research synthesis* can be applied to all kinds of knowledge, this discussion is limited to some examples of how the synthesis of health sciences research literature has evolved. The practices and tools used today for reviewing the health sciences literature can be traced back to 1879 with the publication of Index Medicus, a medical bibliography that included a subject and author index to articles published in medical journals.[3] Today's most useful tools, however, are relatively recent innovations. An historical awareness of how the research literature has grown and when some of these tools were introduced will help put these developments into perspective.

Since the mid-1940s, the number of scientific publications has increased dramatically. What spurred this increase is complicated and best left to social and medical historians to explain, but certainly a major factor has been a concomitant rise in the amount of funding for research by the National Institutes of Health (NIH). These growth rates are shown in Figure 1-1. In this example, publications are those defined by the Science Citation Index as original substantive articles, editorial materials, letters, reports of meetings, correction notes, and reviews for the period from 1945 to 1996.[4,5] The NIH dollars are those allocated for research grants.[6]

Some critics suggest that there is no evidence of an increase in the rate of scientific publications over time, citing the following two reasons for this rationale: (1) the quantity of scientific publications has increased, but the quality has not,[7] and (2) the rate of publications per health scientist has remained the same, but the number of health scientists has increased.[8] Neither argument addresses the fact that an individual health scientist today must cope with an increase in the absolute number of journals and publications that have to be considered when reviewing the literature.

In examining the growth rates in Figure 1-1, the increase in NIH grant dollars may not be as steep as indicated because the figures are actual dollars spent for each 5-year period, unadjusted for inflation. The real rate of growth may be flatter or dip more in some years than others, after inflation has been taken into account. For the sake of argument, however, consider the two rates of growth at their face value, and assume an upward trajectory for both.

What is important is the juxtaposition of the growth in the number of publications, the amount of research funding, and developments in resources for creating a synthesis of the research literature. Examples of these developments over the past 50 years can be assigned to three categories: (1) the establishment of bibliographic databases, (2) the availability of electronic tools for manipulating information, and (3) the emergence of synthesis applications.

## Bibliographic Databases

Bibliographic databases include information in print and electronic form. The first major development in this category for the health sciences was the creation of the National Library of Medicine (NLM) under the aegis of the Public Health Service of the Department of Health, Education, and Welfare. The NLM evolved from the Library of the Army Surgeon General's Office, which was established in 1836.[3] With major

## Figure 1-1

Developments in research synthesis compared with number of scientific publications and funding for research grants from the NIH. *Source:* Data about publications are from Science Citation Index 1945–1954 Cumulative Comparative Statistical Summary, in *SCI Science Citation Index Ten Year Cumulation 1945–1954: Guide and Lists of Source Publications,* pp. 18–19, © 1988, Institute for Scientific Information; and Comparative Statistical Summary 1955–1996, in *SCI Science Citation Index 1996 Annual Guide and Lists of Source Publications,* pp. 57–63, © 1997, Institute for Scientific Information. Data about NIH research funds are from NIH Almanac 1997, in Branch EO, Publication No. 97-5, 1997, National Institutes of Health.

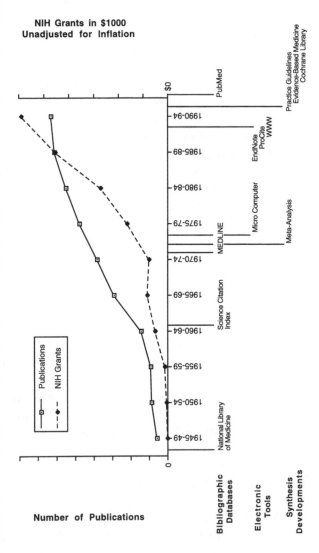

funding from Congress in 1942, the NLM gathered together a national collection of scientific books, papers, and reports located in Washington, DC. Accessing this information electronically was difficult for scientists in other parts of the country; this was only partially solved in 1961 with the creation of the Science Citation Index and later its sister application, the Social Science Citation Index, by Eugene Garfield, PhD.[9] These indexes are owned and published by the Institute for Scientific Information, which was acquired by Thomson Scientific in 1992. In 1971, MEDLINE, an electronic database of the scientific literature in medical and other health-related journals and publications, was launched by the NLM and became one of the premier tools for the health sciences researcher. Initially, access to MEDLINE was brokered by reference librarians, which made frequent or spontaneous use awkward in the daily life of most scientists. Such use could also be expensive; a charge per reference had a chilling effect on financially strapped graduate students and unfunded assistant professors—the very users who most needed such access.

The rules for searching MEDLINE were also complicated. Reference librarians had to undergo specialized training in order to master the intricacies of the search, and not all research libraries had specialized personnel. Nonetheless, the availability of an electronic database that could be searched to locate specific studies was a major advantage for the health scientist engaged in research synthesis.

Gradually, an infrastructure for an electronic bibliographic database became more refined, with standardized key words and more easily understood rules for creating a search strategy. Although scientists intent on using the electronic version of MEDLINE were still bound to one of the research libraries, and bound even more tightly to the services of a knowledgeable librarian, this ability to access the research literature was a major advantage. The number of research publications had already begun an upswing by this point in time. This is reflected in the rate of growth shown in Figure 1-1 for the period after MEDLINE became available, although cause and effect have not been clearly established between the development and the rate.

The period since MEDLINE's inception has seen the creation of a myriad of other bibliographic databases, such as PsycINFO, International Pharmaceutical Abstracts, and CINAHL. Two additional bibliographic databases were launched around the turn of the 21st century— PubMed in 1997 and PubMed Central in 2008. PubMed, based in the

National Library of Medicine, provides worldwide access to MEDLINE on the Internet. Anyone—scientist or layperson—now has access to the MEDLINE database of over 18 million references just by signing onto its website. Not only is PubMed free, but the use of MEDLINE is no longer tied geographically to a library or restricted to the availability of a qualified librarian. All that is needed is a computer and access to the Internet.

PubMed Central, a part of the National Institutes of Health, is a free, digital archive of biomedical and life sciences literature. The goal of PubMed Central is to provide full-text papers, not just abstracts, of scientific research funded by the NIH. These two databases, PubMed and PubMed Central, are interrelated, and together provide rapid and often complete access to research publications.

## Electronic Tools

Only a few examples of developments in the second category, that of electronic tools, are described, beginning with the microcomputer. Without a doubt, the introduction in the mid-1970s of a reasonably priced personal computer represents a seminal event in any historical description of the late 20th century. For the reviewer of the literature, the availability of a personal computer vastly improved the quality of a scholarly life. Word processing software, together with information in bibliographic databases, made the tasks of searching and abstracting the scientific literature far more efficient.

There continued to be other problems, however, one of which was the lack of a standardized format for citations and references to articles in scientific journals or books. If a health scientist had to switch from one formatting system to another in the preparation of a paper or report, then he or she was forced to go back through the entire document and make the changes one by one. Although there is still no single, universal format, another kind of solution was developed. In the late 1980s, two reference management software packages were produced that made changes from one formatting system to another automatically, thus providing some relief for the time-strapped researcher. Academicians created both software products. EndNote was introduced in 1988 and ProCite in 1989. RefWorks, introduced in 2002, is a Web-based product that is generally available to faculty and students through an institutional subscription from university and college libraries. Not only do these software packages satisfy their original intent of allowing the user to switch from one reference formatting system to another, but they now have additional features such as the creation of a reference library on the user's own computer or Web-based document, a search and sort capability, a seamless download of a reference and its abstract from electronic bibliographic databases to desktop computers, and the flexibility of user-defined information for each reference.

The impact of reference management software packages does not equal that of the personal computer in a list of important developments in the history of research synthesis or information management. Nevertheless, these software products are good, solid tools for everyday use and are like a set of well-honed kitchen utensils compared with the discovery of fire—the latter is necessary, but after that is available, the former makes the job easier.

Like the personal computer, another advance comparable to the discovery of fire was the establishment of the World Wide Web in 1989. With the Web, individual researchers have the capability of free and unlimited worldwide access to information, not only among each other, but also to banks of information such as the electronic bibliographic databases and other scientific forums that have rapidly proliferated. The use of these electronic tools in combination with bibliographic databases, together with an increase in the absolute number of scientific publications and NIH grant dollars, contributed to developments in the third category of development—that of synthesis applications.

## Synthesis Applications

It is easy to imagine that if the same rate of growth in scientific publications had been seen in the financial market, investors would have been ecstatic. There was more research, better science, and an exponential growth in new information, but the scientific community pondered how to make use of it. How could this growing reservoir of scientific knowledge be managed and used for the betterment of humankind or, at least, for individual patients? Three developments in the late 1990s illustrate a response to these issues: practice guidelines, evidence-based medicine, and the Cochrane reviews of clinical trials. These developments are shown at the far right of the timeline in Figure

1-1. Before their appearance, however, a new methodological technique, meta-analysis, was proposed in the mid-1970s, just before personal computers and the Web became available.

## Meta-Analysis

A professor of education, Gene Glass, was one of the first to outline a way of statistically summarizing the results of multiple studies on the same topic. His initial paper was published in 1976.[10] Health scientists quickly saw the advantage of this technique and began to apply it to biomedical research studies. The use of this and other techniques contributed to the development of the following prime examples of synthesis applications in the 1990s:

- Clinical practice guidelines generated largely by the Americans
- Evidence-based medicine created by the Canadians
- Reviews by the worldwide Cochrane Collaboration led by the British

All of these resulted from national and international collaborations, made possible by local, national, and international funding. These developments depend on the resources of bibliographic databases, electronic tools, and an intense commitment to making use of available research findings to improve the health care of the individual and the public.

## Clinical Practice Guidelines

Practice guidelines were developed with the intention of providing practitioners, such as physicians, nurses, and allied health professionals, with sound strategies based on the scientific literature for delivering the best possible health care. A formal definition of a clinical practice guideline was provided by the Institute of Medicine in 1992.[11]

In 1993, the first Practice Guideline was commissioned and funded by the Agency for Health Care Policy and Research (AHCPR), a federal granting agency created by Congress in 1989. Over the following five years, AHCPR commissioned practice guidelines on 19 topics that were published between 1992 and 1998. Examples of topics include acute pain management, depression in primary care, HIV infection, otitis media with effusion in children, and poststroke rehabilitation.

In conjunction with the American Association of Health Plans and the American Medical Association, AHCPR developed the National Guideline Clearinghouse website, http://www.guideline.gov, dedicated to enhancing access to the guidelines in 1998. Currently, the successor of AHCPR (the Agency for Healthcare Research and Quality) has redefined its role as that of facilitator to other organizations such as specialty societies or managed care organizations or local groups of clinicians in their development of future practice guidelines.

## Evidence-Based Medicine

The basic concepts of evidence-based medicine were conceived by a group of academicians at McMaster University in Hamilton, Ontario, led by Professor G. H. Guyatt. The medical school at McMaster has long been known for its innovativeness in medical education, and these clinician-scholars expanded their audience from a classroom of medical students in southern Canada to healthcare providers throughout the world.

Guyatt and his colleagues recognized the need for members of the medical community to improve their ability to evaluate and use the scientific literature.[9] An ongoing series of users' guides, published in *JAMA*, has provided a set of tutorials for clinicians on such diverse topics as how to use articles about diagnosis, prognosis, grading health care recommendations, and applicability of clinical trial results. A list of such articles from 1993 to 2000 is provided in Appendix A.[12-44] The concepts of evidence-based medicine have been adopted by clinicians in other disciplines, including nursing, dentistry, and pharmacy. A term with broader application has begun to emerge, that of *evidence-based practice*. The relationship between evidence-based practice and clinical practice guidelines has not been fully examined, although, logically, they are closely linked. Clearly, what they have in common is a foundation of scientific literature that has been carefully reviewed and systematically abstracted. At its simplest, evidence-based practice is what a practitioner such as a physician or nurse-clinician does one-on-one with a patient, whereas practice guidelines provide guidance for best clinical practice.

## The Cochrane Collaboration

An example of a more recent development of a synthesis application is that of the Cochrane Library, an electronic library of systematic reviews of the clinical literature created and maintained by the Cochrane Collaboration.

In 1992, a nonprofit organization, the Cochrane Centre, was created in Oxford, England, in response to concerns expressed 20 years earlier by Archie Cochrane, a British epidemiologist.[45] An outgrowth of the Centre was the establishment in 1993 of the Cochrane Collaboration, an international, voluntary, collaborative effort to provide systematic and critical reviews of randomized, controlled trials of health care.[46] Participants in the collaboration are organized through collaborative review groups that include researchers, healthcare professionals, and consumers throughout the world, including experts in the United States and Canada.

The ongoing mission of the Cochrane Collaboration is to prepare, maintain, and promote the accessibility of systematic reviews of the effects of healthcare interventions. Current information about the Cochrane Collaboration can be found at http://www.cochrane.co.uk.

The Cochrane Collaboration is an example of the international, multidisciplinary nature of the current field of research synthesis. Communication is rapid and easily accessible via the Internet. Lay audiences can readily obtain information available in the Cochrane Library. Thus, the Cochrane Library has an important role to play in the democratization of healthcare information. The availability of the Cochrane Library dates back to the mid-1990s. The further development and impact of this resource for health professionals, policy makers, and consumers bear close scrutiny in the future.

This brief history of the emergence of the field of research synthesis in the health sciences has focused exclusively on developments in English language systems, and largely in North America, with some mention of the role of the British. Linguistic and geographic boundaries of science are disappearing daily, however, and the full scope of developments and use of research synthesis cannot be confined to a single language or these few countries. Globalization exists in the scientific arena, including the private sector.

In the future, the history of research synthesis will need a broader cultural and linguistic perspective in order to provide a complete understanding of the impact of this discipline on the health of people. The role of the Internet, the importance of multidisciplinary collaboration, and access to scientific knowledge by people who are not health professionals will also be important factors in understanding how research synthesis can have an impact on the health and lives of people throughout the world.

For the present, the surfeit of information in the health sciences literature presents both a challenge and an opportunity. A systematic way of conducting a literature review incorporating the efficient use of those resources is needed. The Matrix Method offers one such system.

# THE MATRIX METHOD: DEFINITION AND OVERVIEW

The Matrix Method is both a structure and a process for systematically reviewing the literature. The structure is provided by the Lit Review master folder that contains all of the notes and documentation you accumulated as you reviewed the literature. The Lit Review master folder includes four other folders, as shown in Exhibit 1-1, consisting of the following:

1. **Paper Trail Folder—Keeping Track of Where You Have Been**. This is a record of the search process used to identify relevant materials. Examples include notes about the materials examined, key words used to search the electronic bibliographic databases in the library, and instructions for electronic searches. Think of this as a chronologic diary or personal blog about the process you went through as you conducted this review of the literature.
2. **Documents Folder—Organizing Documents for Review**. This section includes a downloaded copy, pdf file, or link of the journal articles, book chapters, and other materials gathered for your review of the literature. These are the documents used to create a review matrix, which goes in the third folder.
3. **Review Matrix Folder—Abstracting Each Document**. The review matrix is a spreadsheet or table with columns and rows that you use to abstract selected information about each journal article, book chapter, or other materials included in your review of the literature.
4. **Synthesis Folder—Writing the Review of the Literature**. This is the outcome of your use of the Matrix Method, a written synthesis of your critical review of the literature based on the materials you abstracted in the review matrix.

In addition to structure in the form of a lit review master folder, the Matrix Method also provides a process for how to create and use the

| Exhibit | |
|---|---|
| **1-1** | **Structure of the Matrix Method: Sections of the Lit Review Master Folder** |

| Type of folder | Purpose |
|---|---|
| • Paper Trail folder | Keeping track of where you've been |
| • Documents folder | Storing documents for review |
| • Review Matrix folder | Abstracting each document |
| • Synthesis folder | Writing the review of the literature |

materials in each of the four folders. That process is described in Chapters 3 through 6. The Matrix Method was specifically designed for reviews of the health sciences literature, but it can be used for reviews of the literature in any field by anyone at any level of expertise, from novice to seasoned reviewer. The key to the versatility of the Matrix Method lies in the use of the review matrix, which is described briefly here and is explained in greater detail in Chapter 5.

In the two previous editions of this book, a lit review book was described as a three-ring notebook with four sections. This was a hard copy approach to creating and using the Matrix Method. With the third edition, however, the Matrix Method has been converted to an electronic system through the use of a master folder and four separate folders within it. If you want a hard copy approach, then locate an earlier edition of this book. If that's not possible, then substitute a three-ring notebook for the master folder, and create four sections with tab dividers, one each for the four types of folders in Exhibit 1-1.

# REVIEW MATRIX: A VERSATILE TOOL

With a review matrix, you create a structured abstract of all of the source documents from your literature review. A review matrix is like a spreadsheet or table—a rectangular arrangement of columns and rows. All that is needed to set up a blank review matrix is a blank spreadsheet or the table option in a word processor.

The columns across the top of a review matrix are the topics or headings you use to abstract each document or study. The rows down the page are the documents or studies. The point at which each column and row meets is a cell, which is where you write notes about a document. An example of the format for a review matrix is shown in Exhibit 1-2, in which there are four columns and two rows. Each column has a topic, such as author/title/journal, year, purpose, or type of study design, and each row consists of a journal article. Thus, the review matrix is a place to record notes about each article, paper, study, or report on the basis of a standard set of column topics.

Column topics can range from the very general to the specific. For example, a review matrix for Shakespeare's plays might include these column topics: setting, characters, protagonist, antagonist, and psychological theme. Alternatively, if the focus was on the scientific literature, the matrix would feature other kinds of column topics: hypothesis, independent variables, dependent variable, methodological design, and sampling design.

No matter the level of expertise or area of focus, you are entirely in control of the review matrix. You decide which column topics to use and which documents or studies to review. The process you use to make those decisions—which topics, which documents—is described in this book. In the course of making those decisions, abstracting the articles, and writing the synthesis, you begin to take ownership of the literature.

| Exhibit | | | | |
|---|---|---|---|---|
| **1-2** | **Example of the Format of a Review Matrix** | | | |
| | **Column 1** | **Column 2** | **Column 3** | **Column 4** |
| | Example: | Example: | Example: | Example: |
| | **Author, title, journal** | **Year** | **Purpose** | **Type of study design** |
| Row 1 | | | | |
| | Journal article 1 | 1995 | Drug treatment for epilepsy | Experimental study |
| Row 2 | | | | |
| | Journal article 2 | 1997 | Drug treatment | Case-control study for depression |

# OVERVIEW OF CHAPTERS AND APPENDICES

The creation and use of the review matrix and lit review master folder are described in the remaining chapters. Although the Matrix Method can be applied to the literature on just about any topic, there is an emphasis throughout this book on the health sciences. The nine chapters in this book are organized into the following three parts:

- Part I. Fundamentals of a Literature Review—Chapters 1 and 2
- Part II. The Matrix Method—Chapters 3 through 6
- Part III. Applications Using the Matrix Method—Chapters 7 through 9

Chapters 2 through 9 are described briefly here, followed by an overview of the Appendices. At the end of each chapter is a section titled "Caroline's Quest," which includes practical examples of how the concepts can be applied.

## Chapter 2: Basic Concepts

This chapter consists of definitions of concepts that are fundamental in any review of the literature, especially those used in the Matrix Method. Also included in this chapter is a description of the different parts of a typical scientific paper published in most health-related journals. If you know where to find specific topics, then you will be in a better position to abstract the study. Chapter 2 also describes the basic elements of a methodological review of the literature. These elements can be used as the sole basis of a review, or more realistically, as a list of possibilities for inclusion, together with the content of the field under review. A list of potential column topics for reviewing the research methodology in the scientific literature is given in the section "Guidelines for a Methodological Review of the Literature."

## Chapter 3: Paper Trail: How to Plan and Manage a Search of the Literature

This chapter describes what steps to take in doing a review of the literature, how to develop a key words list, how to locate source materials, how to use the snowballing technique, what to consider in a computer search of established databases such as MEDLINE, PsycINFO, and Science Citation Index, and use of the Internet.

## Chapter 4: Documents Folder: How to Select and Organize Documents for Review

This chapter includes a description of how to choose documents and organize journal articles and other source materials. The advantages of maintaining a chronologically ordered set of pdf files or other types of electronic copies in the Documents folder are also discussed.

## Chapter 5: Review Matrix: How to Abstract the Research Literature

The review matrix is the heart of the Matrix Method. This chapter describes how to set up a review matrix, including issues such as choosing topics to abstract, variations in topics, addition of topics later in the process, and a step-by-step guide for constructing the review matrix.

## Chapter 6: Synthesis: How to Use a Review Matrix to Write a Synthesis

This chapter is a description of how to use the review matrix to critically analyze and write a review of the literature, including a discussion of differences between a summary and a synthesis.

## Chapter 7: A Library of Lit Review Master Folders

This chapter describes the advantages of maintaining a collection of lit review master folders for use over time, or by a team of people, or across interrelated topics. Specifics include how to create and expand a library of lit review master folders.

## Chapter 8: The Matrix Indexing System

This chapter describes a system for integrating information from electronic databases and reference libraries created with reference management software and copies of papers in the Documents folder in the Lit Review master folder. The advantages of this system are discussed, together with information about how to set up and use such a system.

## Chapter 9: Matrix Applications by Health Sciences Professionals

This chapter describes four kinds of applications for the experienced health sciences professional. These include the use of the Matrix Method in (1) conducting a research project, from writing a grant proposal to publishing the results; (2) standardizing the review process for a meta-analysis; (3) creating and using clinical practice guidelines; and (4) applying the concepts of evidence-based medicine.

## Appendix A: Useful Resources for Literature Reviews

This is a handy list of books, journals, and Internet websites that can be useful in searching further for scientific literature that is not available in the standard sources. The appendix is a potpourri of useful information.

## Appendix B: Structure of Computer Folders for the Matrix Method

This appendix describes how to create and organize computer folders on your desktop for the Matrix Method. Examples are given to help you understand this structure before you use the Matrix Method to review the literature.

# REFERENCES TO WEBSITES

Website addresses are given throughout the remaining chapters and especially in Appendix A. Each address on the Internet, called a universal resource locator (URL), was examined and determined to be accurate and functional at the time this book went to press; however, the Internet is a dynamic environment, and URLs can change on an hourly basis. For this reason, neither the author nor the publisher is responsible for the accuracy of the URLs provided in this book.

# Caroline's Quest: Understanding the Process

Just as a picture can be worth a thousand words in explaining a concept, a practical example can be equally valuable in demonstrating a process. With that in mind, each of the nine chapters in this book will conclude with a description of the experiences of a typical graduate student, Caroline Collins, as she learns about matrix applications and uses the Matrix Method and the Matrix Indexing System in reviewing the literature on smoking behavior for her master's thesis in public health. Caroline's thesis topic was the characteristics of teenage girls who smoke.

Caroline tends to be a bit impatient and will occasionally try to take shortcuts in order to avoid some of the more time-consuming details of the Matrix Method. Fortunately, she meets weekly with her advisor, Professor Dickerson, who gives her advice about using the Matrix applications. Caroline's experiences and Professor Dickerson's explanations illustrate not only the process but also the rationale for why certain steps in the Matrix Method are needed and how the Matrix Indexing System can help her organize her materials.

In medieval times, a quest was a chivalrous enterprise involving an adventurous journey that often required courage or determination. In modern times, a quest is defined as a search or pursuit. Although Caroline does not have to deal with dragons in the library, her review of the literature does require persistence and determination in her pursuit of knowledge—a pursuit that is occasionally adventurous. Thus, in both the modern and the ancient senses of the word, Caroline has embarked upon a quest.

# REFERENCES

1. Russell CL. An overview of the integrative research review. *Progress in Transplantation*. 2005; 15 (1): 8–13.

2. Oxman AD, Cook DJ, Guyatt GH, for the Evidence-Based Medicine Working Group. How to use an overview. Users' guides to evidence-based medicine. *JAMA*. 1994;272(17):1367–1371.

3. National Library of Medicine. Images from the history of the Public Health Service: Biomedical research. U.S. Department of Health and Human Services, Public Health Service; 2005. http://www.nlm.nih.gov/exhibition/phs_history/100.html/. Accessed November 1, 2005.

4. Institute for Scientific Information. Science citation index 1945–1954 Cumulative comparative statistical summary. In: *SCI science citation index ten year cumulation 1945–1954: Guide and lists of source publications*. Vol 8. Philadelphia, PA: Institute for Scientific Information; 1988:18–19.

5. Institute for Scientific Information. Comparative statistical summary 1955–1996. In: *SCI science citation index 1996 Annual guide and lists of source publications*. Vol 1. Philadelphia, PA: Institute for Scientific Information; 1997:57–63.

6. National Institutes of Health. *NIH almanac 1997*. Washington, DC: NIH Publication No. 97–5; 1997.

7. Garfield E. In truth, the "flood" of scientific literature is only a myth. *Scientist*. 1991;5:11–25.

8. Huth EJ. The information explosion. *Bull NY Acad Med*. 1989;65:647–661.

9. Garfield E. *The index with all the answers*. Thomson Scientific. Available at: http://scientific.thomson.com/promo/celebration/sci. Accessed November 1, 2005.

10. Glass G. Primary, secondary, and meta-analysis of research. *Educational Researcher*. 1976;5:3–8.

11. Fields, MJ, Lohr N, eds. *Guidelines for clinical practice: From development to use*. Washington, DC: Institute of Medicine; Division of Health Care Services; 1992.

12. Guyatt GH, Rennie D. Users' guides to the medical literature. *JAMA*. 1993;270:2096–2097.

13. Oxman AD, Sackett DL, Guyatt GH. Users' guides to the medical literature: I: How to get started. *JAMA*. 1993;270:2093–2095.

14. Guyatt GH, Sackett DL, Cook DJ, for the Evidence-Based Medicine Working Group. Users' guides to the medical literature. II: How to use an article about therapy or prevention. A: Are the results of the study valid? *JAMA*. 1993;270:2598–2601.

15. Guyatt GH, Sackett DL, Cook DJ, for the Evidence-Based Medicine Working Group. Users' guides to the medical literature. II: How to use an article about therapy or prevention. B: What were the results and will they help me in caring for my patients? *JAMA*. 1994;271:59–63.

16. Jaeschke R, Guyatt GH, Sackett DL, for the Evidence-Based Medicine Working Group. Users' guides to the medical literature. III: How to use an article about a diagnostic test. B: What are the results and will they help me in caring for my patients? *JAMA.* 1994;271:703–707.

17. Jaeschke R, Guyatt G, Sackett DL, for the Evidence-Based Medicine Working Group. Users' guides to the medical literature. III: How to use an article about a diagnostic test. A: Are the results of the study valid? *JAMA.* 1994;271:389–391.

18. Laupacis A, Wells G, Richardson WS, Tugwell P, for the Evidence-Based Medicine Working Group. Users' guides to the medical literature. V: How to use an article about prognosis. *JAMA.* 1994;272:234–237.

19. Levine M, Walter S, Lee H, et al. Users' guides to the medical literature. IV: How to use an article about harm. *JAMA.* 1994;271:1615–1619.

20. Oxman AD, Cook DJ, Guyatt GH, for the Evidence-Based Medicine Working Group. Users' guides to the medical literature. VI: How to use an overview. *JAMA.* 1994;272:1367–1371.

21. Guyatt GH, Sackett DL, Sinclair JC, et al. Users' guides to the medical literature. IX: A method for grading health care recommendations. *JAMA.* 1995;274: 1800–1804.

22. Hayward RS, Wilson MC, Tunis SR, Bass EB, Guyatt G, for the Evidence-Based Medicine Working Group. Users' guides to the medical literature. VIII: How to use clinical practice guidelines. A: Are the recommendations valid? *JAMA.* 1995; 274:570–574.

23. Richardson WS, Detsky AS, for the Evidence-Based Medicine Working Group. Users' guides to the medical literature. VII: How to use a clinical decision analysis. B: What are the results and will they help me in caring for my patients? *JAMA.* 1995;273:1610–1613.

24. Richardson WS, Detsky AS, for the Evidence-Based Medicine Working Group. Users' guides to the medical literature. VII: How to use a clinical decision analysis. A: Are the results of the study valid? *JAMA.* 1995;273:1292–1295.

25. Wilson MC, Hayward RS, Tunis SR, Bass EB, Guyatt G, for the Evidence-Based Medicine Working Group. Users' guides to the medical literature. VIII: How to use clinical practice guidelines. B: What are the recommendations and will they help you in caring for your patients? *JAMA.* 1995;274:1630–1632.

26. Naylor CD, Guyatt GH, for the Evidence-Based Medicine Working Group. Users' guides to the medical literature. XI: How to use an article about a clinical utilization review. *JAMA.* 1996;275:1435–1439.

27. Naylor CD, Guyatt GH, for the Evidence-Based Medicine Working Group. Users' guides to the medical literature. X: How to use an article reporting variations in the outcomes of health services. *JAMA.* 1996;275:554–558.

28. Drummond MG, Richardson WS, O'Brien BJ, Levine M, Heyland D, for the Evidence-Based Medicine Working Group. Users' guides to the medical literature. XIII: How to use an article on economic analysis of clinical practice. A: Are the results of the study valid? *JAMA.* 1997;277:1552–1557.

29. Guyatt GH, Naylor CD, Juniper E, et al. Users' guides to the medical literature. XII: How to use articles about health-related quality of life. *JAMA*. 1997;277: 1232–1237.

30. O'Brien BJ, Heyland D, Richardson WS, Levine M, Drummond MF, for the Evidence-Based Medicine Working Group. Users' guides to the medical literature. XIII: How to use an article on economic analysis of clinical practice. B: What are the results and will they help me in caring for my patients? *JAMA*. 1997;277: 1802–1806.

31. Dans AL, Dans LF, Guyatt GH, Richardson S, for the Evidence-Based Medicine Working Group. Users' guides to the medical literature. XIV: How to decide on the applicability of clinical trial results to your patient. *JAMA*. 1998;279:545–549.

32. Barratt A, Irwig L, Glasziou P, et al. Users' guides to the medical literature: XVII: How to use guidelines and recommendations about screening. JAMA. 281: 2029–2034; 1999.

33. Bucher H, Guyatt G, Cook D, Holbrook A, McAlister F, for the Evidence-Based Medicine Working Group. Users' guides to the medical literature. XIX: Applying clinical trial results. A: How to use an article measuring the effect of an intervention on surrogate end points. *JAMA*. 1999;282:771–778.

34. Guyatt G, Sinclair J, Cook D, Glasziou P, for the Evidence-Based Medicine Working Group and the Cochrane Applicability Methods Working Group. Users' guides to the medical literature. XVI. How to use a treatment recommendation. *JAMA*. 1999;281:1836–1843.

35. McAlister F, Laupacis A, Wells G, Sackett D, for the Evidence-Based Medicine Working Group. Users' guides to the medical literature. XIX: Applying clinical trial results. B: Guidelines for determining whether a drug is exerting (more than) a class effect. *JAMA*. 1999;282:1371–1377.

36. Randolph AG, Haynes RB, Wyatt JC, Cook DJ, Guyatt GH, for the Evidence-Based Medicine Working Group. Users' guides to the medical literature. XVIII: How to use an article evaluating the clinical impact of a computer-based clinical decision support system. *JAMA*. 1999;282:67–74.

37. Richardson WS, Wilson MC, Guyatt GH, Cook DJ, Nishikawa J, for the Evidence-Based Medicine Working Group. Users' guides to the medical literature. XV: How to use an article about disease probability for differential diagnosis. *JAMA*. 1999;281:1214–1219.

38. Giacomini MK, Cook DJ, for the Evidence-Based Medicine Working Group. Users' guides to the medical literature. XXIII: Qualitative research in health care. B: What are the results and how do they help me care for my patients? *JAMA*. 2000;284:478–482.

39. Giacomini M, Cook D, for the Evidence-Based Medicine Working Group. Users' guides to the medical literature. XXIII: Qualitative research in health care. A: Are the results of the study valid? *JAMA*. 2000;284:357–362.

40. Guyatt GH, Haynes RB, Jaeschke RZ, et al. Users' guides to the medical literature. XXV: Evidence-based medicine: Principles for applying the users' guides to patient care. *JAMA*. 2000;284:1290–1296.

41. Hunt D, Jaeschke R, McKibbon K, for the Evidence-Based Medicine Working Group. Users' guides to the medical literature. XXI: Using electronic health information resources in evidence-based practice. *JAMA*. 2000;283:1875–1879.

42. McAlister F, Straus S, Guyatt G, Haynes R, for the Evidence-Based Medicine Working Group. Users' guides to the medical literature. XX: Integrating research evidence with the care of the individual patient. *JAMA*. 2000;283:2829–2836.

43. McGinn T, Guyatt G, Wyer P, et al. Users' guides to the medical literature. XXII: How to use articles about clinical decision rules. *JAMA*. 2000;284:79–84.

44. Richardson WS, Wilson MC, Williams JW Jr, Moyer VA, Naylor CD, for the Evidence-Based Medicine Working Group. Users' guides to the medical literature. XXIV: How to use an article on the clinical manifestations of disease. *JAMA*. 2000;284:869–875.

45. Cochrane A. *Effectiveness and efficiency: Random reflections on health services.* London, England: Nuffield Provincial Hospitals Trust; 1992.

46. Chalmers I. The Cochrane Collaboration: Preparing, maintaining and disseminating systematic reviews of the effects of health care. *Ann NY Acad Sci.* 1993;703:156–163.

# 2 Basic Concepts

In this chapter, we review concepts fundamental to a review of the literature. Then we describe the structure of a typical research paper published in a scientific journal in order to clarify where information can be found. This chapter consists of the following sections:

- ⊙ Source Materials Defined
- ⊙ Different Kinds of Source Materials
- ⊙ Anatomy of a Scientific Paper—Finding What You Need in a Typical Research Paper
- ⊙ Guidelines for a Methodological Review of the Literature
- ⊙ Caroline's Quest: Learning the Concepts

# SOURCE MATERIALS DEFINED

Source materials are publications and other documents about scientific knowledge that are analyzed in a review of the literature. Examples include papers published in scientific journals, reference books, or chapters in books, textbooks, and reports published by governmental and nongovernmental agencies and organizations.

# DIFFERENT KINDS OF SOURCE MATERIALS

## Primary, Secondary, and Tertiary Source Materials

An understanding of the differences between primary, secondary, and tertiary source materials is important in selecting documents for a literature review.

- *Primary source materials* are original research papers written by the scientists who actually conducted the study. An example of primary source material is the description of the purpose, methods, and results section of a research paper in a scientific journal by the authors who conducted the study.

  A review of the scientific literature is based on the assumption that primary source materials have been examined and analyzed, unless otherwise noted. You handicap yourself if you do not use primary source materials because the details of a study may be missing from or misinterpreted in a summary about the study. Alternatively, secondary and tertiary source materials might prove to be very useful in the search for relevant primary source materials.

- *Secondary source materials* are papers or other documents that summarize the original work of others. In other words, secondary source materials are based on information from primary source materials. Although secondary source materials often are written by individuals other than those who actually did the research, it is possible for authors to summarize their own previously published or reported research, in which case, these later summary descriptions can still be considered secondary source materials.

Examples of secondary source materials include a summary of the literature in the introduction of each scientific research paper published in a journal, a description of what is known about a disease or treatment in a chapter in a reference book, or the synthesis you write as you review the literature.

- *Tertiary source materials* consist of a systematic analysis or critical review of scientific papers. The boundaries between secondary and tertiary source materials are not hard and fast; rather, they merge from one into another and differ in the degree of critical and systematic analysis as the review moves from secondary to tertiary. The term itself has not been standardized.

The availability of tertiary source materials has evolved over the past 25 years. With the veritable explosion of scientific knowledge and the rapid rise in the number of new sources, scientists and practitioners alike have been forced to not only stay abreast of new information, but also to find more efficient ways to abstract, synthesize, and critically evaluate that knowledge. Tertiary source materials provide a variety of ways to accomplish the task of qualitative and quantitative evaluation of research findings.

Often, tertiary source materials have a specific focus. Examples include papers or articles such as a critical review of all randomized clinical trials on a subject such as the reviews in the Cochrane Library, a meta-analysis, practice guidelines, or papers that support evidence-based medicine. Each of these types of tertiary source materials is described more fully in Chapter 3.

## Publications

Traditionally, source materials have been published in books or scientific journals that assume a permanence of documentation and are usually publicly accessible through libraries. This format has changed in recent years to include journals published in electronic form on the Internet. For example, Internet resources include primary source papers in peer-reviewed scientific journals and secondary source documents such as those in the annual reviews. Regardless of how the results of a scientific study are communicated, a basic requirement of source materials is public accessibility. Not all materials that are publicly accessible are free. There may be a charge, depending on the source. Proprietary materials (those owned by individuals or organizations for their exclusive use), secret documents (such as those marked "classified" by the government), and confidential reports that cannot be accessed by people outside of a company or without a security clearance generally are not used as source materials in published, peer-reviewed journals. In other words, if you have access to such materials but those who read your review do not, then those restricted materials probably should not be included in a review of the literature.

## Peer Review

Modern scientific inquiry carries the twofold assumption that knowledge is built on previous thought, and the methods and results of research are documented and available for all to inspect and study. A basic expectation of a paper describing original research, especially in scientific journals, is that it has been evaluated through the peer-review process. A peer is a person with the same (or superior) expertise in a scientific subject as the author of a research article. A peer-reviewed paper is one that has undergone the scrutiny of one or more scientific experts. Although peer review provides one kind of quality control in the scientific process, it is not the only measure of scientific quality, nor is it a guarantee of excellence. People who read the scientific literature must decide for themselves whether each study meets the standards of the research community. A review of the literature provides one way of comparing studies and assessing the excellence of each study as well as the body of research on a specific topic. *Ulrich's Periodical Directory* (available in both print and electronic forms) is a good source to determine whether a journal is peer reviewed.

## Scientific Abstracts

A scientific abstract is an abbreviated description of a study or theory. Abstracts of papers presented at scientific meetings are considered source materials, although they usually do not include enough information about the research methods to permit a reviewer to make a judgment about the scientific merit of the study. Abstracts often are restricted in length and format—for example, no more than 250 to 500 words—and usually are without citations of other research papers. For this reason, some journals, such as the *Journal of the American Medical Association*, do not permit the inclusion of references to abstracts in a summary of the review of the literature in peer-reviewed journal articles. An example of an abstract presented at a professional meeting is shown in Exhibit 2-1.

For purposes of reviewing the literature, however, abstracts of papers from scientific meetings can be useful in several ways, for example, by

- Alerting the reviewer to the more recent scientific studies
- Providing useful leads to discovering other, more fully described studies
- Identifying the name and location of researchers who can be contacted for further information

In many fields, abstracts of papers presented at scientific meetings are included in a special issue of the journal published by the society or organization that sponsored the meeting. Alternatively, the abstracts may be issued in booklet form or in CD-ROM format at the conference.

| Exhibit | |
|---|---|
| **2-1** | **Example of an Abstract in a Journal** |

### DRUG USE MANAGEMENT IN BOARD AND CARE FACILITIES

*J. Garrard, S.L. Cooper, C. Goertz*

*Abstract* The purpose of this study was to describe medication management in board and care facilities throughout Minnesota. A triangulation of data collection methods was used, including mail questionnaires (N = 98 facilities), telephone interviews (N = 64 facilities), and site visits (N = 15 facilities). Major issues examined included characteristics of board and care facilities, staffing, residents, and drug management systems. Results showed that staff in 86% of the board and care facilities surveyed provided medication storage, 83% gave medication reminders, and 69% administered medications to one or more residents. Site visits revealed a wide diversity in the characteristics of managers and their attitudes toward medication administration.

In this case, the abstracts might be available to only those who attended the meeting. Contacting the author or someone who attended the meeting may be the only way of obtaining a copy of the abstracts. Recently, some professional and scientific societies have begun to publish on the Internet a list of titles or abstracts of papers presented at national or international meetings. This possibility could be explored by searching the Internet for the website of the professional society and then determining whether the abstracts are available. A list of professional societies and their websites is provided in Appendix A.

## Citations, References, Bibliographies

A citation provides documentation about the source of an idea, statement, or research study referred to in a written document. Citations occur in the text or body of a scientific paper or book. In and of itself, a citation provides very little actual information; you have to go to the list of references or the bibliography (usually at the end of the paper or chapter in a book) in order to find out more about the document being cited, such as the title of the paper or the journal that it was published in or the year of publication.

Different formats for citations are used, depending on the preference of the journal or book. Two common formats are numerical and author's last name. In the numerical format, the citation is given at the end of the cited material (usually at the end of a sentence) as a superscript number. In the author's last name format, the citation, usually located at the end of the sentence, is given as the authors' last names and the year of publication, enclosed in parentheses. These and other examples can be found in a style manual such as *Elements of Style*.[1] Examples of the numerical and author's last name formats are shown in Exhibit 2-2.

A reference is the actual documentation of the work cited and should provide the information needed to find the work referred to. References are usually located at the end of a scientific paper or chapter in a book. See the end of this chapter for an example. The references of some documents, such as government reports or congressional records, are sometimes hard to decipher, and a reference librarian can be helpful in locating these materials.

Many different formats have been devised for the listing of references, and these differences have caused headaches for generations of

| Exhibit | |
|---|---|
| **2-2** | **Examples of Formats of a Citation in a Research Paper** |

*Numerical Format:* These and other examples can be found in a style manual such as Elements of Style.[26]

*Author's Last Name Format:* These and other examples can be found in a style manual such as Elements of Style (Strunk & White, 1979).

students and researchers in the health sciences. Style manuals such as those by the American Psychological Association[2] and the American Medical Association[3] can be used.

In writing your own papers, including a review of the literature, there are also computer software programs, such as EndNote, ProCite, and RefWorks, that can be used to automatically convert a list of references into the correct format depending on which style you choose. Those resources are described more fully in Chapter 8. Examples of two of the most common formatting styles used in listing references are shown in Exhibit 2-3. These two examples, numerical and author's last name, correspond to the citations shown in Exhibit 2-2.

A tutorial that covers how to cite both print and electronic formats in American Psychological Association, Modern Language Association,

| Exhibit | |
|---|---|
| **2-3** | **Examples of Formats for References** |

**General Format**

Authors. (Year of publication). *Name of Book.* City, State: Publisher.

**Examples**

*Numerical Format:*

26. Strunk W Jr, White EB. *The Elements of Style.* New York, NY: MacMillan; 1979.

*Author's Last Name Format:*

Strunk, W., Jr., & White, E. B. (1979). *The elements of style.* New York, NY: MacMillan.

and Turabian/Chicago styles is available at http://tutorial.lib.umn.edu/infomachine.asp?moduleID510.

Formatting rules for citations and references to printed materials are fairly well known; however, similar rules for sources on the Internet have emerged only recently. Consult the style manuals about how to cite sources on the Internet.

A bibliography is similar to a list of references, except that it also includes references to books and other documents not quoted or cited in the text but are suggested for further reading. Authors often recommend additional materials for readers to consult if they want to develop a better understanding of the subject. Most scientific journals, however, do not encourage or allow bibliographies; these journals limit the writers to lists of references cited in the text.

In summary, the distinctions between a citation, a reference, a list of references, and a bibliography can be described as follows:

- A *citation* is used in the body of a document to give credit to the publications of others or the author's previous work.
- A *reference* for that citation gives complete information about where to find the materials, including the title of the scientific paper, the name and volume number of the journal, and the year published. A reference is usually located at the end of a scientific paper.
- A *list of references* consists of all of the references that were cited in a scientific paper and is usually given at the end of a paper or book chapter.
- A *bibliography* consists of not only references but also other books or papers that provide additional information about the subject being discussed. Most scientific journals restrict authors to references rather than bibliographies.

# ANATOMY OF A SCIENTIFIC PAPER— FINDING WHAT YOU NEED IN A TYPICAL RESEARCH PAPER

## Overview

Knowing where to find something is often as important as knowing what to do with it after you have found it. Thus the first step in conducting a review of the literature is to understand the basic format or structure of a scientific paper.

Research articles, especially those published in scientific journals, are the most common type of source materials used in reviews of the scientific literature. Most research articles follow a standard structure, which is described in this section. By knowing this structure, you can more easily locate different parts of the research study to abstract.

In describing the eight sections of a research paper in a typical scientific journal, some additional comments have been included that might be useful to consider.

> These extra comments are set aside in boxes so they can be easily skipped by people with more experience in reading the scientific literature.

## Title/Authorship Section

The first section consists of the title of the paper and name and affiliations of the author or authors who conducted the research and wrote the paper.

> The order of the authorship is important in most journals, with the first author usually being the person who had the most responsibility for the research paper. In some fields, the most senior scientist is listed last in order of authorship. This is often the person who provided the research mentorship, the laboratory, or the grant support for the research being reported; however, he or she may not have taken the primary responsibility for the study being published. Knowledge of the field itself is needed to determine whether this protocol is followed in the peer-reviewed journals in a particular field.

## Abstract Section

The abstract section includes a brief summary of the paper. Although often identical in length and format to the abstract of a paper presented at a scientific meeting, the abstract section at the beginning of a scientific paper is just one part of the study described more fully in the remainder of the article.

> Summarizing the abstract section of selected journal articles does not constitute a review of the literature because there are usually not enough details in this brief description to allow you to understand how the research was done or how to interpret the results.

## Introduction Section

Generally, the introduction section includes the following four major parts: (1) a brief summary of the authors' review of the literature, (2) the motivation for the paper (i.e., what is missing or unknown in the research literature up to the time the study began), (3) an overview of the scientific theory or conceptual models on which the research was based, and (4) the purpose of the research study described in this paper. Depending on the journal or the author, the purpose of a study can be in the form of a statement, a research question, or a hypothesis.

> Sometimes, authors seem to forget what their original purpose was (whether it was explicitly stated or not), especially in light of interesting results that may have answered another unstated research question. Alternatively, authors may have satisfied the purpose they stated but then asked and answered additional research questions as the paper progresses. You have to decide for yourself whether the authors described a complete purpose in the introduction section of their paper and presented results about the purpose they stated in the introduction section.

## Methods Section

The methods section is a description of the procedures used to carry out the research study and should be complete enough to permit another researcher to replicate the study without the need to contact the authors. The methods section of a typical scientific paper includes information on methodological design, subjects, data sources, data collection methods, and statistical and analytical procedures.

*Methodological Design.* This describes how the research was structured, including the use of pretesting and posttesting, the use of one or more groups of subjects (e.g., experimental and control groups), and how subjects were assigned to these groups, for example, random assignment by the researcher or self-selection into groups by subjects of the study. This subsection should also include a description and definition of each of the major variables in the study, including the independent and dependent variables and the covariates. Some studies will not have an independent variable or a covariate, but all have one or more dependent variables.

*Subjects.* This is a description of how the subjects were chosen for the study—the inclusion and exclusion criteria, sampling design, and number of subjects included in the study and their characteristics, such as gender, age, and disease status. This subsection may also include a description of how many individuals were initially selected; the number who actually participated in the study; and differences between those chosen, those who agreed to participate, those who dropped out, and those who participated at each stage of the research.

*Data Sources.* This subsection is an explanation of whether the information about the subjects in the study was based on primary source data, secondary source data, or both. Primary source data are gathered by the researchers who are reporting the study; secondary source data are gathered by others.

Secondary source data should not be confused with secondary source materials as described at the beginning of this chapter. If secondary source data are used, then the authors should include a description of the characteristics of the database; the original reason the data were gathered, for example, as administrative records or as claims files for healthcare reimbursement; and the dates during which the data were gathered. Some studies will include both primary and secondary source data, for example, information from a survey of the subjects by the researchers, which the same researchers then combined with clinical data obtained from the medical charts that were recorded by the treating physicians.

*Data Collection Methods.* This is a description of all of the procedures used in primary source data collection to gather information from or about the subjects in the study. In this subsection of a journal article, the questionnaire, survey, interview protocol, or other data collection instrument is described, including either the results of validity and reliability analyses of the data collection instrument or references to other studies that include such information.

*Statistical and Analytic Procedures.* This subsection describes the types of statistical tests or analytical procedures used and the assumptions underlying their use, if applicable.

Not all research papers published in health-related journals will include these five subsections in a methods section, and even if they are included, they may not be in the order described previously. Also, a method not described in the methods section may be mentioned later in the results section.

The choice and order of subsections in the methods section of a scientific paper depend on the field, the content, the type of study, and the choices made by the individual author.

The appearance of a previously unannounced set of methods in the results or discussion section may suggest a lack of tidiness in the authors' style of reporting. Alternatively, such a practice may be entirely appropriate if the results of the main research question suggested to the researchers that they should explore something further and the methods for that exploration are then described.

## Results Section

The results section gives the results of the study and in so doing answers the research question, verifies or refutes the hypothesis, or addresses the purposes of the study that should have been stated in the introduction section. This may be the shortest section of the entire paper, and the details may be presented concisely in one or more tables or figures.

> The results section may also require the most intensive reading in order to understand the findings fully. Some journals limit this section only to results; others allow authors to discuss their interpretation of the findings in this section. If interpretations are included, you must be sure to distinguish the actual results from the authors' interpretations or opinions.

## Discussion/Conclusion Section

The discussion/conclusion section usually addresses these five areas:

1. *Summary* of the research study as it relates to the purpose or research question or hypothesis described originally.
2. *Interpretation* and discussion of what these results mean. This is the part of the paper in which the authors can express their opinions about the interpretation of the findings.
3. *Description* of the strengths and weaknesses of the study, including methodological strengths and weaknesses.
4. *Discussion* of future research. Often the results of one study suggest additional research questions. A brief description of these topics may be included in this section of the paper.
5. *Statement* about the significance of this research study on the field. This is not statistical significance, but rather a description about the impact of the findings.

> As with other parts of a research paper, this discussion/conclusion section may not include all of these topics or be in the same order, and there may also be other topics not included in this discussion.

## List of References

The list of references is a listing of all of the papers or other sources cited by the authors in describing previous or related research.

## Acknowledgments Section

This section includes a description of how the research study was funded, for example, the names of granting agencies or foundations and names of individuals who assisted in the research or review.

In summary, the first step in reviewing a scientific paper in a research journal is figuring out where things are, and the eight topics in this section provide a framework for doing that. The second step is understanding what research methods the authors used to carry out their study. The next section describes some fundamentals about research methodologies used in many of the health-related journals.

# GUIDELINES FOR A METHODOLOGICAL REVIEW OF THE LITERATURE

## Overview

A review of the literature can be done from a number of different perspectives, such as variations in the theories on which the studies were based, the hypotheses tested, or the research results. Reviews can also include an examination of the research methodology that constitutes the framework of most empirical studies. In this section, guidelines for abstracting the research methodology of studies in the health sciences are described. Using these methodological guidelines will not only help you analyze what the authors did, but these guidelines will also let you determine what they did not do.

As described previously, most papers published in scientific journals in the health and behavior literature follow a standard format: introduction, methods, results, and discussion. Usually, the methods section of a journal article includes information about how the study was designed and analyzed. Exhibit 2-4 is an outline of methodological topics described in this section.

| Exhibit | |
|---|---|
| **2-4** | **Methodological Topics for Reviewing Research Studies in the Health Sciences Literature** |

Purpose of the paper
Method
  Research design
  • Operational definition of variables
  • Independent and dependent variables
  • Intervention
  • Methodological design
  • Random assignment
  Data collection instruments and procedures
  • Data sources
  • Data collection designs
    —Pre-post design
    —Prospective/retrospective
    —Longitudinal/cross-sectional
  • Data collection instruments
    —Author-designed instruments
    —Standardized instruments
    —Other instruments
  • Instrument characteristics (number of items, format)
  • Psychometric characteristics of data collection instruments
    —Validity studies about the instrument
    —Reliability studies about the instrument
  • Setting
  Subjects
  • Unit of analysis
  • Selection criteria, including inclusion and exclusion criteria
  • Random selection of subjects
  • Sampling design
  • Subject characteristics
  • Number of subjects
    —Participation and attrition rates
    —Participant/nonparticipant differences
  Data analysis
  • Statistical methods
  • Statistical assumptions
Results
Discussion/conclusion
  • Interpretation of results
  • Strengths and weaknesses
  • Significance of results (practical or clinical)
  • Conclusions
References
Acknowledgments

Admittedly, the list in Exhibit 2-4 may seem ambitious as a potential outline of what to abstract about the research methodology. To include all of these topics in a review of the literature, in fact, would be excessive. This is only a set of suggestions, and it is up to you to decide which are relevant to your review.

## Purpose

It is best to begin by asking yourself what the purpose of the study was. Why did the authors do this particular study? What was their purpose or hypothesis or research question? Distinguish between what they said (or implied) their purpose was in the introduction section of the paper and what they actually addressed or answered in the results section.

> The authors may describe the purpose in the form of a general statement, a hypothesis, or a research question. A mark of poor research quality is a paper that does not state specifically the purpose of the study in the introduction section.

## Methodology

In reviewing the methodology, consider how the authors carried out the study. For a review of elements as they are used in the social and behavioral sciences, see the book by Neuman[4] and its counterpart for epidemiological research methods by Kleinbaum and colleagues.[5] Some major topics to consider for methodology follow.

## Operational Definition of Variables

How were the variables in the study operationally defined (i.e., what procedures or steps did the researchers use to measure the variables of interest)? For example, how did they operationally define health or quality of life or education?

## Independent and Dependent Variables

Specify the independent and dependent variables. Describe the independent variable in terms of what was actually done to the experimental group (the intervention in some studies) and to the control group. The dependent variable is the outcome variable.

## Intervention

Describe the procedures or treatment applied to one or more of the groups of subjects, usually to the experimental group, including the timing of the procedures with respect to data collection. Sometimes these intervention procedures are summarized as part of the methodological design.

Depending on the purpose of the research, some studies may not include an actual intervention. Alternatively, the intervention may be some external event, such as a change in health policy or a formulary change, and the purpose of the study is to examine the effects of such a change. In these kinds of studies, the author is expected to give a clear description of the externally applied intervention. Sometimes such a description is not given because it is so well known in the field; if this is the case, there should be at least a reference to a book or journal article or other document or source material that does describe the well-known intervention.

An example of an intervention is a diabetes education program presented to the experimental subjects but not to those in the control group. Sometimes interventions are not applied by the researchers themselves. For example, an intervention might be a federal regulation such as a restriction on the use of antipsychotic medications in nursing homes. In this example, the nursing homes in the experimental group may have been under the federal regulation, and those in the comparison group of homes may not be operating under the regulation.

Finally, some studies may not have an intervention at all, and there may be only one group of subjects. In that case, there is no independent variable, although there should definitely be a dependent variable. There may or may not be covariates, depending on the research question.

## Methodological Design

What was the study design? In the behavioral sciences, the four major designs include experimental, quasiexperimental, preexperimental, and observational. In epidemiologic terms, similar designs are used but are described in different terms. Some examples include randomized control trials, case-control studies, cohort designs, and descriptive designs. Qualitative designs such as those that use focus groups would also be listed here.[6] See the texts by Campbell and Stanley[7] and Cook and Campbell[8] for a description of the behavioral sciences designs. Kleinbaum et al.[5] describe the epidemiological designs.

## Random Assignment

How were the subjects of the study assigned to the experimental and control groups? If the assignment was random, then random assignment was used. If subjects could choose for themselves which groups to be in or if they were already in groups to begin with (such as smokers and nonsmokers), then random assignment was not used.

Technically, the term *experimental design* implies the use of random assignment of subjects to groups, but recent usage has become a bit lax. You need to ask yourself whether the authors specifically said that the subjects were randomized, or randomly assigned, if they said they used an experimental design. A general rule is that if the authors knew enough about methodological designs to randomly assign subjects to groups, then they should have known enough to brag about it in the methodology section.

Also, bear in mind that there is a big difference between random assignment and random sampling. The purpose of random assignment is to create two or more subject groups that are as equal as possible at the beginning of an experimental study, that is, before an intervention is applied. Usually, one of these groups is designated as the experimental group; the other is the control group. Random assignment is a methodological design issue. Random sampling is concerned with the selection of a representative sample of subjects from a population.

## Data Collection Instruments and Procedures

This group of topics is concerned with how information was collected. Examples include data collection procedures, such as questionnaires, surveys, and administrative or clinical records. In this section, the methods themselves should also be described, for example, use of focus groups,[8] the Delphi technique, or an interview protocol that the researchers developed. Some basic reference books that might be useful include those on questionnaire design,[9] conducting a survey,[10] and the design and use of focus groups.[6]

### Data Sources

As described earlier in this chapter, primary source data consist of information gathered by the researchers who conducted the original study from subjects in that study. Alternatively, data gathered by others or for purposes other than research are called secondary source data.

Secondary source data can come in many forms. Some examples include information gathered for administrative purposes (e.g., in registering people when they are admitted to a hospital) or for reimbursement of healthcare services or to document the effects of treatment. If secondary source data were used, note why the data were collected initially (e.g., health services claims files or as part of administrative records).

Another example of secondary source data gathered for purposes other than research includes information collected about a patient's symptoms by clinicians in a medical center and recorded in a clinical record. If a researcher is interested in using that information in a study of those patients, then he or she would be using secondary source data. On the other hand, if the researcher surveys the patients directly about their symptoms, then the data would be primary source data.

An example of a national secondary source dataset is the National Health and Nutrition Examination Survey, which is a national survey about the health and nutritional status of Americans conducted by the National Center for Health Statistics. The initial survey was conducted in the early 1960s.

In some studies, data from different sources are combined to create a database, and these data sources can be from primary or secondary sources or both. For example, a researcher interested in the effects of a specific drug on the cognitive status of older patients may use a medical evaluation questionnaire to gather primary source data from patients and then use data from the patients' insurance company to gather additional information about healthcare costs. In this example, the two data sets, primary and secondary, would be linked through an individual identifier such as the patient's name or code number.

## Data Collection Designs

Begin by noting when the data were collected, for example, "pre-post-post" for one pretesting and two posttestings, that is, one testing before the intervention and two testings after the intervention. Also determine whether the data were gathered prospectively or retrospectively. Were the data gathered at two or more points in time (possibly a longitudinal study) or at a single point in time (cross-sectional)? If primary source data were used, what specific data collection methods or instruments were used to collect information? For example, was the information gathered by questionnaire, survey, telephone, or in-person interview?

## Psychometric Characteristics of Data Collection Instruments

For each data collection instrument, note whether the author describes results of validity and reliability testing of the data collection instrument. If the author developed the instruments but no information was given about validity and reliability, then make a note of the lack of information about these fundamental psychometric characteristics.

In the language of data collection, an *instrument* can be a questionnaire or a list of interview questions, sometimes called a "protocol," or a set of instructions for recording certain behaviors about subjects by the person observing those subjects. For example, a questionnaire might consist of questions about different kinds of foods, and the subject is asked to check off each food he or she ate. An interview protocol is generally a set of questions that the researcher asks. The wording and the order of the questions are both important, and the interviewer usually is not allowed to deviate from that order.

Psychometrics is the study of the characteristics of tests or data collection instruments, including the validity and reliability of the instrument. Validity concerns whether the data collection instrument measures what it was intended to measure. Reliability generally is concerned with stability over time. If researchers want to measure change in the health of a group of subjects, then they do not want an instrument that varies, either in the way it is used or interpreted (validity) or in its consistency each time it is used (reliability). Researchers want a stable data collection instrument to use in studying behavior of their subjects, which may vary over time or across individuals. In other words, any variation the researcher sees should be due to changes in the subjects, not in the instrument itself.

## Instrument Characteristics

Other basic characteristics about a data collection instrument might include the number of items or questions or the average time needed to gather the information from individual subjects. If the instrument was a survey, note whether the data were collected by mail, telephone, or the Web.

Some journals permit the author to publish an author-developed survey as an appendix at the end of the journal article; if such a survey has been included, indicate this in your notes.

### Standardized Instruments

If the instruments were standardized, what references are given about this standardization? What normative groups were used in the original standardization, and did the subjects in this study have the same or similar characteristics as those in the normative group? For example, the norms for a questionnaire about food preferences may have been based on responses from people living in rural Minnesota, but such normative responses might not be appropriate for Chinese Americans living in San Francisco.

### Setting

If relevant to the area of research being reviewed, note the setting in which the data were collected, for example, urban or rural, community, hospital, or nursing home, home, or school.

## Subjects

Summarize the key features about the subjects of the research study.

### Unit of Analysis

What was the unit of analysis? Generally, there are four choices: individual, group, organization, and social artifact.

Examples of the different units of analysis are the following:

- *Individual.* The subject of the study is an individual person. For example, in a study of smoking behavior of teenage children, the child would be the unit of analysis.
- *Group.* The subject is a group of people. For example, in a study of the relationship between family size and group cohesiveness, the family would be considered the unit of analysis.
- *Organization.* The subject is an organization such as a health department or school or hospital. For example, a study of health departments throughout the United States that do or

do not have staff assigned to develop prevention programs for AIDS would use the health department as its unit of analysis.

- *Social artifact.* A social artifact has been defined in the research literature as the product of a social being. Examples of social artifacts include a healthcare policy or law or practice guideline. An example of research in which a social artifact was the subject would be a study of the characteristics of state guidelines on vaccination of preschool children. Thus, the state guideline (which is a social artifact) would be the unit of analysis for this study.

Most, but not all, studies in the health and behavioral sciences use the individual as the unit of analysis. If another unit of analysis was used, then it is important to determine how the researchers operationally defined that unit. For example, if an organization, such as a hospital, was the unit of analysis, then did the researchers define what they meant by a hospital in terms such as bed size, geographic area, or type of ownership? In this example, record the role of the individual who spoke on behalf of the hospital, such as the chief financial officer or the medical director.

## Selection Criteria

What were the inclusion and exclusion criteria used to select subjects?

An example of inclusion criteria might be age range and type of health plan; only people between the ages of 18 and 64 years and who were enrolled in a managed health care organization qualified for a study. Thus, people whose ages were less than 18 years or older than 64 years and/or those who had some other kind of health care plan were excluded from the study.

## Random Selection and Sampling Design

How were subjects selected for this study? Did the researcher select the subjects, and did he or she select them randomly from a population of potential subjects? If the subjects volunteered for the study, then they were not randomly selected. These are very important points to note because the generalization of results to a population is not technically possible without random selection.

Under this topic, you should also note which sampling design was used. Some examples include simple random sample, stratified random sample, cluster sample, and convenience sample.

> Sometimes researchers do not describe the sampling design they used. Read the article carefully to see whether you can figure this out from their description of what they did. An excellent book on sampling designs is the one by Kish.[11]

## Subject Characteristics

Which subject characteristics did the authors describe? Examples include gender, age (recorded as mean age or percent within age categories or age range), race or ethnicity, or other characteristics such as disease status, geographic location, or socioeconomic status.

## Number of Subjects

How many subjects were in the study? The number of subjects in a study is often abbreviated as $N = x$. For example, in a study with five subjects, they might use ($N = 5$) in tables of results.

> The number of subjects is a fundamental piece of information that some authors fail to provide; therefore, you might consider noting the total number or its absence in every study. If there is more than one group of subjects, for example, an experimental (E) group and a control (C) group, then record the number for each group in this cell, for example: E ($N = 126$), C ($N = 140$).

Summarizing the number of subjects can involve a number of related questions that may be important to your review of the literature.

*Participation and Attrition Rates.* What was the total number of subjects the researchers began with compared with the number who left during the study and the final number of subjects who completed the study? These enumerations can be surprisingly difficult to find in a scientific paper.

*Participant/Nonparticipant Differences.* What information was given about differences between people who stayed in the study and those who either refused to be in the study in the first place or left before the study ended? A similar discussion about participant and nonparticipant differences might be in terms of the dropout rate or respondent and nonrespondent analysis.

Equally noteworthy is the absence of a description of such differences. This is an important issue that concerns the possibility of bias in the final group of subjects for whom data were analyzed.

## Data Analysis

Summarize how the data were analyzed, including the use of descriptive statistics such as percentages or means, a bivariate analysis such as chi-square or *t* test, or multivariate techniques such as analysis of variance or regression analysis.

A basic statistics textbook is a good resource in providing background material for this section. The classic book by Siegel on nonparametric statistics is also useful.[12,13] Statistical methods commonly used in the epidemiological literature include those described in books by Fleiss[14] and Kahn and Sempos.[15]

### Statistical Methods

What specific statistical and other analytic procedures were used in the study (e.g., logistic regression, analysis of variance, factor analysis, and path analysis)? An example of an analytic technique for qualitative research would be a content analysis of interview data.

### Statistical Assumptions

What assumptions (or violation of assumptions) were made by the author about the use of the analytic techniques other than the usual procedures described in introductory texts?

## Results

In analyzing the results of a study, ask yourself the following questions:

- Did the authors answer the research question they posed in the introduction section of the paper? After you have read the entire paper, ask whether this was the right question in the first place.
- Did the authors provide an answer to a research question that they did not ask initially? In other words, did some results creep into the paper without an explicit research question being described? Were these additional research questions appropriate to the study?

A transition from one research question or purpose to another can sometimes be detected in the results section or, more often, in the discussion section of the paper. Such a change usually occurs because the authors allowed the statistically significant results to dictate the hypothesis rather than the other way around. Differences between initial and later research questions may be important to note in a review of the study.

## Discussion/Conclusion

This collection of topics describes the authors' scientific opinions about the study. In reviewing a paper, you need to separate the results of the study, which are facts, from the authors' interpretations or opinions of the results and their significance.

## Interpretation of Results

As a reviewer, it is up to you to decide whether the authors' interpretations are logical and valid based on the results of the study. You must also decide whether the results of this study are consistent with the findings of other studies on the same topic as described elsewhere in the literature.

## Strengths and Weaknesses

What strengths and weaknesses of the study were described? Specifically, did the authors address issues such as whether the findings could be generalized, problems with methodological design that were present but could not have been remedied, sample size adequacy, or sampling design?

> Authors who do not point out the weaknesses of their own studies make themselves vulnerable to such criticisms from others. Most authors are pleased to describe the strengths of their studies; some may be a bit reluctant to discuss the weaknesses.

## Conclusion

When reviewing this section, describe what the authors concluded from this study. Note especially whether the conclusions and the significance of the findings related to the results. Do you agree with those conclusions? Bear in mind that statistical significance does not always result in clinical significance or a meaningful impact.

# Caroline's Quest: Learning the Concepts

"So," Caroline looked at Professor Dickerson somewhat challengingly, "isn't the Matrix Method just a spreadsheet that's called a review matrix?"

"No," he replied, "there's more to it than that. The Matrix Method is a system for how you can access, integrate, and use information from a variety of sources in order to prepare a written synthesis of the scientific literature. In the past, researchers could keep up with the current literature by reading several journals or monitoring the work of a few well-known scientists in a field, or they could simply call or write their friends who did research in that area."

"What's wrong with doing that now?" Caroline asked. This business of accessing and integrating and so forth was beginning to sound rather time consuming as she thought about all the other things she had to do to get her thesis completed. She asked, "Why bother with the Matrix Method?"

Professor Dickerson looked over the top of his glasses at her and said dryly, "Because the amount of scientific literature has grown tremendously. It's rarely possible to develop a comprehensive understanding about the research literature on a topic by using such informal methods. Fortunately, more advanced tools for searching and accessing the literature have become available over the past decade or so. The Matrix Method takes advantage of those tools."

"But no one else in my program has to go to all this trouble for their lit reviews," Caroline complained. Her voice verged on the edge of a whine as she continued, "They just go to the Web, read a few papers, and write up a summary. Takes them several hours at most."

Professor Dickerson nodded his head, "Yes, anyone can do a sloppy job, Caroline." He again looked over the top of his glasses at her. "But they run the risk of not understanding the literature—neither the depth nor the full scope of what's out there. Furthermore, they could miss some of the more important articles or even major trends in a field of research. It is also the case that whatever they write, whether it's a thesis, a scientific paper, or whatever, has to withstand the scrutiny of readers who are likely to know the literature quite well . . . like your thesis committee members."

Caroline's eyes were beginning to glaze over as he continued, "The person who does a cursory literature review could find himself doing what he thinks is original research, only to discover at the end that that very study was already done and reported previously by someone else."

Professor Dickerson's enthusiasm began to build. "The process of doing a thorough review of the literature is analogous to solving a mystery. If you miss some of the important clues, then you may not ever find out who or what was responsible for the crime—or what the study really meant, in this case. The Matrix Method gives you a systematic way to lay out all of the pieces and put the puzzle together."

He looked at her with a grin. "The effort will pay off for you, Caroline. You'll see. Now, let's get started."

Under Professor Dickerson's direction, Caroline created a lit review master folder on the desktop of her computer and assigned four folders to the master folder. She further subdivided the first folder, Paper Trail, into five parts, with one document, to begin with, for each part. The different sections and subsections of Caroline's Lit Review master folder are shown in Exhibit 2-5.

She then went to the biomedical library to begin by looking up some reference books on smoking behavior. In her opinion, just using Google to search for the topic would have been sufficient, but Professor Dickerson insisted that she read from the original textbooks as her first step.

| Exhibit | |
|---|---|
| **2-5** | **Outline of Caroline's Lit Review Master Folder for Her Thesis Topic** |

Paper Trail folder
- Key words
- Key sources
- Electronic bibliographic database
- Internet
- Notes

Documents folder
Review Matrix folder
Synthesis folder

# REFERENCES

1. Strunk W, White EB. *Elements of Style.* New York, NY: Macmillan; 1979.
2. American Psychological Association. *Publication Manual of the American Psychological Association.* 4th ed. Washington, DC: APA; 1994.
3. Iverson C. *American Medical Association Manual of Style: A Guide for Authors and Editors.* 9th ed. Baltimore, MD: Williams & Wilkins; 1998.
4. Neuman WL. *Social Research Methods: Qualitative and Quantitative Approaches.* 3rd ed. Boston, MA: Allyn & Bacon; 1997.
5. Kleinbaum DG, Kupper LL, Morgenstern H. *Epidemiologic Research: Principles and Quantitative Methods.* New York, NY: Van Nostrand Reinhold; 1982.
6. Krueger RA. *Focus Groups: A Practical Guide for Applied Research.* Thousand Oaks, CA: Sage Publications; 1994.
7. Campbell DT, Stanley JC. *Experimental and Quasi-Experimental Designs for Research.* Chicago, IL: Rand McNally; 1966.
8. Cook TD, Campbell DT. *Quasi-Experimentation: Design and Analysis Issues for Field Settings.* Chicago, IL: Rand McNally; 1979.
9. Salant P, Dilman DA. *How to Conduct Your Own Survey.* New York, NY: John Wiley & Sons; 1994.
10. Dillman DA. *Mail and Telephone Surveys: The Total Design Method.* New York, NY: John Wiley & Sons; 1978.
11. Kish L. *Survey Sampling.* New York, NY: John Wiley & Sons; 1995.
12. Siegel S. *Nonparametric Statistics for the Behavioral Sciences.* New York, NY: McGraw-Hill; 1956.
13. Siegel S, Castellan NJ. *Nonparametric Statistics for the Behavioral Sciences.* 2nd ed. New York, NY: McGraw-Hill; 1988.
14. Fleiss JL. *Statistical Methods for Rates and Proportions.* New York, NY: John Wiley & Sons; 1981.
15. Kahn HA, Sempos CT. *Statistical Methods in Epidemiology.* New York, NY: Oxford University Press; 1989. *Monographs in Epidemiology and Biostatistics,* vol 12.

Part

# II The Matrix Method

# 3

# Paper Trail: How to Plan and Manage a Search of the Literature

This chapter discusses how to set up and use a paper trail and how to organize and conduct a search for source materials in your review of the literature. The five sections of this chapter are the following:

- ⊙ What Is a Paper Trail?
- ⊙ How to Create a Paper Trail
- ⊙ How to Find Source Materials: Creating and Using a Paper Trail
- ⊙ Tips on Searching for Source Documents
- ⊙ Caroline's Quest: Managing the Search

# WHAT IS A PAPER TRAIL?

For the purposes of the Matrix Method, a paper trail is a record of lists and notes to help in planning and in keeping track of what you have done as you review the literature on a particular topic; it is a method of documenting your search for relevant materials.

## Advantages of a Paper Trail for You

A paper trail is both a map of where you are going and a diary of where you have been in your search for source documents. The map gets you started and buys you efficiency; the diary helps you remember what you have done so that you can avoid redoing the same thing. Even people with a prodigious memory will find themselves backtracking and trying to relocate materials if they have not taken the time to make a list of the sources explored and the articles considered. It is also useful to write down the names of people who were (or were not) helpful. A knowledgeable and enthusiastic librarian can be worth his or her weight in gold—record the person's name for future reference. The same advice applies to helpful faculty and colleagues.

# HOW TO CREATE A PAPER TRAIL

## Getting Organized

Just as you unfold a map as the first step in going on a hike in unfamiliar territory, the first step in beginning a review of the literature should be to set up a paper trail folder in your Lit Review master folder. At its simplest, a list on a word processing document of topics to be considered will suffice. Although index cards may be traditional, they are not as useful in the Matrix Method as a computer. Some topics to consider for your paper trail folder follow.

## Set Up a Paper Trail Folder

Begin by setting up a paper trail folder with five word processing documents, one for each of the following topics.

1. **Key Words Document**
   A key word is a term or phase that describes a research topic. In this document, keep a list of key words that you have used as well as others that you have considered but discarded.

   Begin the key words document by typing the purpose of the review of the literature at the top of the page. Think of the words that describe that topic. For example, if it is a review of the literature on the epidemiology of pneumonia, some of the key words might be pneumonia, nursing homes, elderly.

   As you collect information during the literature review, add to this list. Some of the terms considered initially may not be useful as the literature review progresses. Leave these terms on the list, but enter a strikethrough or otherwise mark them differently—it is useful to know which terms did not work as well as those that did.

2. **Key Sources Document**
   The key sources document is another list that consists of the names of reference books, journals, government reports, and other materials that you considered or reviewed. The same logic of maintaining a list of where you are going and where you have been applies to all of the library sources considered or explored. For example, in the key sources part of the Paper Trail folder, create a document where you record a running list of reference books, other books, journals, other print sources, bookmarks on the Web, and electronic bibliographic databases.

3. **Electronic Bibliographic Databases Document**
   In the electronic bibliographic databases document, make a list of electronic databases used, such as MEDLINE, CINAHL, and PsycINFO. What were the search strategies? Include the key words used, as well as restrictions on the search, such as English language journals only or review articles only. Include the period of time covered, for example, 1965 to the present. Insert in this section a copy of the results of searches of the electronic

bibliographic databases, such as MEDLINE, including the search strategies used to generate the list of references.

4. **Internet Document**

When researching on the Web, it is easy to lose track of what has been explored unless you keep a record. Do that in this subsection. Also, set bookmarks in your browser for commonly used websites. Another possibility is to copy the URL of the home page of a useful website and put it in the Internet document.

5. **Notes Document**

*Practical Notes.* This is a miscellaneous document in the paper trail. Treat it like a running diary of things that you need to remember. Make notes about where to find hard-to-locate materials, for example, *"Journal of Scientific Wonder* is located in the third stack from the left in the basement of the library of the county medical examiner." The notes refer to the search process, not the papers themselves.

Also, use this subsection to record additional references of scientific papers or other source materials discovered in the process of looking at other sources. Put a check mark by each as you read and accept or discard it. In recording a reference, use a standard format in order to make sure that you have all needed information, including publisher, dates, and page numbers. Inevitably, the one article without the year of publication will be the very one that is essential in your synthesis of the literature. It is best to be consistent in the first place. Examples of standard formats are shown in Chapter 2; choose the reference format of a journal you use frequently.

*Record All Authors.* In recording a reference to a paper in a journal, consider the following tip. Scientific journals are expensive to produce, and editors are inclined to be stingy with space. One way some publishers have of saving space in the references section of a book or journal article is to restrict the names of multiple authors to the first three individuals followed by et al. for the remaining authors. In reviewing these papers, however, you might want to depart from this protocol by writing down the names of all of the authors in the review matrix. There is a practical reason for doing this. In many fields of study, the research is conducted jointly by a number of scientists. Although the first author of a paper presumably had the most responsibility for writing the paper or doing the study, some of the other authors may have been publishing in the field over a longer period of time. These more established scientists sometimes are listed last in the authorship.

Alternatively, authors of some large, well-established research teams have chosen to list their names alphabetically, signifying equal importance in the contribution of all members of the research team to the study. With either practice, there can be a problem in tracking the work of specific individuals if the format of the reference is limited to the first three authors followed by et al. Consider recording all of the authors' names; usually they are listed on the paper itself. After the paper trail folder is set up, you are ready to begin your search of the literature.

*Clarifying Incomplete Citations.* There will come a point, usually at the end of your patience or right before a deadline, when you will come upon one of your citations that is missing a crucial piece of information such as a date or volume number. PubMed may have a solution for this problem. Go to the PubMed home page (http://preview.ncbi.nlm.nih.gov/pubmed). Under PubMed Tools, select Single Citation Matcher. At that site, you can type in any information that you have about the citation (you do not even have to have the exact title), and PubMed will try to provide you with one or more options that fit your criteria. This is a nifty tool whether you have run out of time or not!

# HOW TO FIND SOURCE MATERIALS: CREATING AND USING A PAPER TRAIL

## Reference Books: Learn Something about the Topic

If you are not familiar with the area or subject of the literature you are reviewing, it is important to take time to learn some of the fundamental information about the disease or issue. Reference books can be especially useful resources at the beginning of a review of the literature in providing an overview of the topic, as well as a potential list of key words. In a biomedical library, these books are often kept on reserve and therefore are readily available. Check with the reference librarian about the major reference books on the topic you want to review. For example, if you are reviewing the literature on treatment of arthritis, then consult a basic medical textbook about arthritic conditions and their treatments before conducting a review of the research literature on arthritis medications.

As you consult a reference book or textbook, develop a list of key words, including the terms those authors used. Maintain a list of the textbooks or reference books examined, and with each, record references of papers and other books mentioned at the end of chapters that relate to your subject. Alternatively, make a digital scan of these source materials, and store them in the notes document in the paper trail folder. Record the names of journals cited frequently in these source materials, whether or not any of the papers are of specific interest. This list of frequently appearing journals will also be useful in the next step: collecting articles from the scientific journals.

If you are already familiar with the subject under review, the most efficient approach might be to launch the search for source documents using your list of key words to run a computer search.

## Key Words and Controlled Vocabulary: Searching the Electronic Databases

In searching for journal articles in most health sciences databases, you can use key words or a controlled vocabulary of key words. Key words are terms that describe the characteristics of a subject you are reviewing. A controlled vocabulary is an organized list of approved terms or key words that indexers of the journal or set of journals used to describe the same journal articles.

### Key Words

Key word searching consists of looking for the occurrence of the word(s) in the title and/or abstract of the article exactly as it is typed in the search box. If the author uses an alternative spelling or synonym for the topic, then there is no guarantee that the article will be retrieved by the key word search. For example, if the author uses the word *tumor* in his/her article and the searcher uses the keyword *cancer*, then there is no guarantee that the search will retrieve that article.

Key word searching can be helpful when you are looking for a new drug or a new procedure that has not yet been introduced into the controlled vocabulary of the database. In such a case, key word searching may be the only effective way of retrieving articles about the topic.

## Controlled Vocabulary

When you use the controlled vocabulary to search the same journals in the same database, then you are using the terms that indexers used when they indexed the articles. The controlled vocabulary in MEDLINE/PubMed is called MeSH (medical subject headings). Most databases provide users with direct access to the controlled vocabulary so that you can determine for yourself whether a given term exists for searching. PubMed offers this access through its MeSH database service. Use your search engine to locate this resource at MeSH Home. For example, the official MeSH heading for *cancer* is the controlled vocabulary term *neoplasms*. It does not matter whether an author uses *cancer* or *tumor* in the text of his or her article; the use of the controlled vocabulary term will guarantee retrieval of all articles on the topic.

## Identifying Controlled Vocabulary in Abstracts

Another way to identify controlled vocabulary terms is to examine the abstracts of articles in electronic bibliographic databases. For example, consider the abstract from PubMed shown in Exhibit 3-1. Three of the five MeSH subject headings have an asterisk: Drug Labeling,* Medicine, Herbal,* and Medicinal/chemistry.* An asterisk indicates the MeSH subject heading is a major focus of the article. To find other citations that had a primary focus on those topics, you would restrict your PubMed search to those asterisked MeSH headings by typing the MeSH heading followed by the qualifier: majr in square brackets: drug labeling [majr].

# Electronic Bibliographic Databases: Many Options, Many Differences

Although MEDLINE was one of the first major electronic bibliographic databases established, numerous other databases that cover different subjects and time periods in the health sciences literature are available,

| Exhibit | |
|---------|---|
| **3-1** | **Abstract in the Citation Display from PubMed** |

1: Arch Intern Med. 2003 Oct 27;163(19):2290-5.                                                    Related Articles, Links

FULL TEXT AT
▶ ARCHIVES OF INTERNAL MEDICINE    ⑤ Find It   UNIVERSITY OF MINNESOTA Twin Cities

**Variations in product choices of frequently purchased herbs: caveat emptor.**

Garrard J, Harms S, Eberly LE, Matiak A.

Divisions of Health Services Research & Policy, School of Public Health, and College of Pharmacy, University of Minnesota, Minneapolis 55455, USA. jgarrard@umn.edu

BACKGROUND: Patients who report use of herbs to their physicians may not be able to accurately describe the ingredients or recommended dosage because the products for the same herb may differ. The purpose of this study was to describe variations in label information of products for each of the 10 most commonly purchased herbs. METHODS: Products for each of 10 herbs were surveyed in a convenience sample of 20 retail stores in a large metropolitan area. Herbs were those with the greatest sales dollars in 1998: echinacea, St John's wort, Ginkgo biloba, garlic, saw palmetto, ginseng, goldenseal, aloe, Siberian ginseng, and valerian. RESULTS: Each herb had a large range in label ingredients and recommended daily dose (RDD) across available products. Strengths were not directly comparable because of ingredient variability. Among 880 products, 43% were consistent with a benchmark in ingredients and RDD, 20% in ingredients only, and 37% were either not consistent or label information was insufficient. Price per RDD was a significant predictor of consistency with the benchmark, but store type was not. CONCLUSIONS: Persons self-medicating with an herb may be ingesting ingredients substantially different from that recommended by a benchmark, both in quantity and content. Higher price per label RDD was the best predictor of consistency with a benchmark. This study demonstrates that health providers and consumers need to closely examine label ingredients of presumably the same or similar herbal products.

MeSH Terms:
- Cross-Sectional Studies
- Drug Labeling*
- Humans
- Medicine, Herbal*
- Plants, Medicinal/chemistry*

PMID: 14581247 [PubMed - indexed for MEDLINE]

*Source:* Reprinted from PubMed, the National Library of Medicine. Abstract adapted with permission by the American Medical Association, 2006. All rights reserved. Garrard, J, Harms, S, Eberly, LE, Matiak, A. Variations in product choices of frequently purchased herbs: caveat emptor. Arch Intern Med 2003, 163(19): 2290–2295.

some of which are listed in Exhibit 3-2. The major database of clinical medicine, MEDLINE, has been freely available over the Internet since 1997 with the National Library of Medicine's PubMed interface. You will find it very instructive to run the same search, using the same key words in two or more of these databases, such as MEDLINE and CINAHL. The databases serve different audiences, and there can be differences in which articles are identified.

After you have generated a list of controlled vocabulary terms and some key words, whether the list is complete, run a search of the literature in whichever electronic bibliographic database you choose (e.g., MEDLINE/PubMed).

In your initial search of the literature in an electronic database, use a search strategy that is as broad as possible. For example, when specifying

| Exhibit | | | |
|---|---|---|---|
| 3-2 | **Examples of Electronic Bibliographic Databases in the Health Sciences** | | |
| **Database** | **Dates covered** | **Subjects covered** | |
| BIOSIS Previews | 1969–present | Biology, biotechnology, biochemistry | |
| CINAHL | 1982–present | Nursing and allied health | |
| CURRENT CONTENTS | Period varies | Multidisciplinary | |
| Digital Dissertations | 1861–present | Abstracts of doctoral dissertations and masters theses from North American universities | |
| Health and Psychosocial Instruments | 1985–present | Measurement instruments in health and behavioral sciences | |
| International Pharmaceutical Abstracts | 1970–present | Pharmaceutical science and practice | |
| MEDLINE | 1966–present | Health sciences | |
| PsycINFO | 1974–present | Psychological literature | |
| Sociological Abstracts | 1963–present | Sociological literature | |

the instructions for an electronic search, include all types of papers, such as editorials or review summaries or letters to the editor, about a particular scientific topic. Even if you do not intend to use such nonempirical communications in your final review of the literature, they may be useful in locating other, more relevant scientific papers that you might not have found otherwise. Editorials and letters to the editor can also be enlightening in suggesting counterpoints or alternative opinions about a study. Finally, these nonempirical communications often include new citations that may be especially useful as you expand your search.

Maintain a copy of database search strategies, that is, the instructions you specify for the electronic search, as well as the complete list of source materials selected. A practical way to do this is to copy the instructions just before initiating the electronic search and then keep a copy in the electronic bibliographic databases document in your paper trail folder. This information may be useful when you check the thoroughness of your search.

A few words of caution: First, conduct the computer search of the literature yourself. This will give you the opportunity to scan a title, consider which authors were involved in the study, or rapidly read the abstract. Such information may be crucial in deciding whether to select the article for further consideration.

In the process of working with the initial results of a computer search, you will begin to pick up subtle cues about what else is in the literature. For example, when scrolling through a list of abstracts by a particular author, you will notice the names of other authors associated with a topic or a journal that often publishes papers in this area. Such information is useful in the later stages of the literature review.

A second cautionary note is to remember that not all journals are included in even the most frequently used databases such as MEDLINE. This is especially true for some of the newer journals or those with a specialized focus. For this reason, it is important to extend your search of the literature to the print versions of some of the scientific journals.

## Scientific Journals: The Most Current Research Literature

In this era of electronic information, it is easier than ever to stay current on new research that is about to be published in the scholarly literature. The days of scanning tables of content or year-end indexes of journals are now past.

PubMed, the NLM's interface to the MEDLINE database, provides access to new research by including publisher-submitted citations to forthcoming articles before publication. These records will be indicated in PubMed with the tag "(PubMed-as supplied by publisher)." These citations can be found in PubMed by searching for a key word, author, or journal title. Publishers can also submit citations that will appear in the electronic (or Web) versions of their publications in advance of the print publication. These citations will appear in PubMed with the tag "(Epub ahead of print)."

Most of these citations will then go through the indexing process and receive a new tag such as "(PubMed-in process)" before being completely indexed for MEDLINE. Not all of these publisher-supplied citations will be indexed for MEDLINE. Other commercial bibliographic database providers of MEDLINE, such as OVID, may include these in-process citations as a separate database. Check with your institution's library to determine whether you have access to these files.

Another way to be notified about upcoming publications is to sign up for e-mail alerts directly from the publisher. Many health sciences journals offer this type of service, and it is usually free. If you sign up for these e-mail alert services, you will receive the table of contents of new issues directly before publication. For example, by searching for *JAMA* using Google, you can find the American Medical Association URL, which will offer you the option of free e-mail alerts of tables of contents of *JAMA* and Archives journals. These include *JAMA*, the *Archives of Dermatology, Facial Plastic Surgery, General Psychiatry, Internal Medicine, Neurology, Ophthalmology, Otolaryngology-Head & Neck Surgery, Pediatrics & Adolescent Medicine,* and *Surgery*. Other journals can be located via Google or one of the other search engines.

## Research in Progress: NIH RePORTER

In reviewing the literature, it is sometimes important to know about studies that are in progress, even if the results are not yet available. For example, if you are thinking about applying for a grant proposal, it is important to find out if a similar study has already been funded. Alternatively, you might have a pressing clinical or patient-related problem for which there is little or no information in the literature, and you need to find out who is doing research on that issue. You may want to identify researchers who have not yet published in an area but who might be presenting results at upcoming scientific meetings. By identifying current research projects, you could follow them in future literature or contact the researchers directly about their plans for publication of results.

Although a list of all research studies ever conducted or even those currently in progress does not exist, you can identify many of the research projects funded by the federal government by conducting a search on the NIH RePORTER. The RePORTER (the RePORT Expenditures and Results module) is part of the larger NIH website, the Research Portfolio Online Reporting Tool (RePORT), at http://report. nih.gov.

This tool was launched in 2009 and is still evolving. It replaces the CRISP query tool by NIH. NIH RePORTER is a searchable database of federally funded biomedical research projects conducted at universities, hospitals, and other research institutions. Projects that have been completed as well as those currently in progress are included in the database.

NIH RePORTER includes studies funded by NIH, the Substance Abuse and Mental Health Services Administration, the Health Resources and Services Administration, the Food and Drug Administration, the Centers for Disease Control and Prevention, Agency for Healthcare Research and Quality (AHRQ), and Veterans Affairs. As of the publication of this book, the URL is http://projectreporter.nih.gov, although this may change as the tool evolves. (Use your search engine to locate NIH RePORTER if this URL fails.)

There are other searchable databases of research grants and clinical trials in specific disciplines. Information about many of these databases can be found at the NLM Gateway (http://gateway.nlm.nih.gov/gw/Cmd?Overview.x). An example of one of the NLM databases is HSRProj, which contains descriptions of research in progress funded by federal and private grants and contracts for use by policy makers, managers, clinicians, and other decision makers. It provides access to information about health services research in progress before results are available in a published form. The HSRProj website is http://wwwcf.nlm.nih.gov/hsr_project/home_proj.cfm.

Another resource is ClinicalTrials.gov (http://www.clinicaltrials.gov), which provides information about randomized clinical trials that are either in progress or are being initiated. The location and a telephone number are provided for the public.

## Government Reports: How to Find Them

Over the past five or more years, different health-related agencies of the federal government have begun to provide special reports on the Internet. A free, searchable database of documents printed by the U.S. Government Printing Office (GPO) is available on the Internet at GPO Access.

Discuss with a reference librarian the search procedures for accessing congressional reports and other federal documents. Many of these materials are not research reports, nor are they necessarily peer reviewed even if they are reports of scientific studies. These documents can be very useful, however, in gathering background material about a topic or issue and suggesting other sources to include in your review of the literature.

An additional Internet resource available on GPO Access is the Government Information Locator Service (GILS), which is a website for finding publicly available federal information resources, including electronic information resources. Use your search engine to locate Government Information Locator Service (GILS).

## Critical Evaluations of the Literature: Critiques by Experts

Increasingly, researcher and practitioner alike are faced with the problem of not only staying abreast of what is new, but also critically evaluating and integrating the results across multiple studies. Although there is no universally agreed on system for synthesizing research studies, different ways of coping with the information explosion have been developed over the past few decades. Four of these strategies are described in this section: (1) review articles, (2) meta-analysis, (3) practice guidelines, and (4) the Cochrane Library.

All four are examples of tertiary source information, as described in Chapter 2; however, there are some major differences among them—some are qualitative and others quantitative; some are guidelines for practitioners, and others are tools for researchers; some are locally focused, and others are international in scope. What they represent, however, are resources that can be explored as you review the literature. Be aware of their existence and consider using them as adjuncts to the usual electronic bibliographic databases.

## Review Articles

In general, a review summarizes or synthesizes what is new or currently known about a topic. Some review articles also provide a critical analysis of the research methods and the quality of the research. Reviews can be found in a variety of print and electronic sources. Some peer-reviewed journals that concentrate on original or primary source papers will periodically publish a review article, such as the 1995 paper, "Alcohol and Mortality: A Review," which was published in the *Journal of*

*Clinical Epidemiology.*[1] In many fields, there are also journals, such as the *Epidemiological Review,* that publish only review articles. Finally, there is a series of annual reviews that has been published since 1932. Currently, these reviews cover approximately 40 disciplines (see a list of these volumes in Appendix A). Further information about these and future volumes can be found at http://www.annualreviews.org.

Even reviews need to be read critically.[2,3] There is a growing literature on criteria for evaluating the quality of reviews for researchers,[3] practitioners,[2] and science writers.[4] In addition, checklists have been developed for what constitutes an acceptable review in the health sciences.[5] An example of a critical review of the quality of reviews in epidemiology is a paper published in 1998, "Quality of Reviews in Epidemiology."[6]

## Meta-Analysis

A meta-analysis consists of a critical evaluation of research studies that statistically combines the results of comparable studies or clinical trials on a specific topic. Unlike review articles, which can be qualitative or narrative in form, a meta-analysis is a statistical tool that can be used to synthesize the findings of different studies quantitatively.

Although a standardized strategy for conducting a meta-analysis has not been accepted, researchers agree on the following procedures:

- *Study protocol.* The analysis must begin with a protocol that states the purpose, methodology, and criteria for selection of studies.
- *Selection of studies.* Primary source papers of empirically based studies, usually experimental studies, must be used.
- *Statistical analysis.* Statistical procedures for combining the results of these studies must be rigorously followed.

There is continuing disagreement about other issues, including the criteria for including and excluding studies with primary source data, whether or not the papers have been published, and whether the data to be analyzed have to be at the study or the individual subject level.[7]

Just as there are criteria for a well-done research study and others for evaluating the quality of a review article, there are also guidelines for a well-done meta-analysis. One set of guidelines was published as a series of articles in the *British Medical Journal* in 1997 and 1998; additional articles are expected to be published in the future.[8-13]

## Practice Guidelines

Clinical practice guidelines were defined in 1992 by the Institute of Medicine, as "systematically developed statements to assist practitioner and patient decisions about appropriate health care for specific clinical circumstances" (p. 2)[14]. Further information is available at the National Guideline Clearinghouse (http://www.guidelines.gov), which is a collection of evidence-based clinical practice guidelines and related documents. The clearinghouse, originally developed by the Agency for Healthcare Research and Quality (AHRQ), the American Medical Association, and the American Association of Health Plans (now America's Health Insurance Plans), is maintained by AHRQ, which is part of the U.S. Department of Health and Human Services.

## Cochrane Library

The Cochrane Library is an electronic library of systematic reviews of health-related research findings produced by the Cochrane Collaboration (http://www.cochrane.org). A standard protocol is used for all Cochrane reviews, as described in the User guides, which can be found by going to the Cochrane Collaboration home page and selecting first-time visitors. The Cochrane Library is rapidly evolving and may eventually become the primary international source of information about the effectiveness of healthcare interventions. This is an important resource for anyone interested in the synthesis of findings about health care interventions across multiple research studies. Cochrane reviews, first released in April 1996, are updated on a quarterly basis and are available by institutional subscription, pay-per-view, or CD-ROM through Wiley Inter-Science. Many university libraries have an institutional subscription to the Cochrane Library; check with the librarian. The abstracts of the reviews are freely available online. Currently, the Cochrane Library consists of seven databases.

1. *Cochrane Database of Systematic Reviews (CDSR)*. CDSR is a collection of systematic reviews of the effects of experimental studies of health care. Each review is prepared by one of the voluntary Cochrane collaborative review groups using preapproved protocols for research synthesis as specified in the Cochrane review

methodology database. The reviews are updated and amended as new evidence becomes available. The CDSR is the primary output of the collaborative. Examples of some of the reviews include the following, as described by the Canadian members of the Cochrane Collaborative based at McMaster University:

- How stroke can be prevented and treated
- Which drugs are effective in the treatment of malaria, tuberculosis, and other infectious diseases
- Which strategies are effective in preventing brain and spinal cord injuries and their consequences

2. *Database of Abstracts of Reviews of Effects.* This contains abstracts of other systematic reviews based on explicit criteria and abstracts from health technology agencies from around the world.

3. *Cochrane Central Register of Controlled Trials.* This is a bibliographic database of randomized clinical trials or experimental studies of healthcare interventions that include trials described in conference proceedings and other sources not usually available in peer-reviewed journals.

4. *Cochrane Database of Methodology Reviews.* This includes publications in journals and books about the science of reviewing research. Also included is a handbook of how to conduct a systematic review and a glossary of terms. The database also describes how to contact the Cochrane Library and information about collaborative review groups.

5. *Cochrane Methodology Register.* This is a bibliography of publications about research methods used in controlled trials from journal articles, books, and conference proceedings. Records include title of the article, where published (bibliographic details), and in some cases, a summary of the article, but not full text.

6. *Health Technology Assessment Database.* This database contains information on healthcare technology assessments, including prevention and rehabilitation, vaccines, pharmaceuticals and devices, medical and surgical procedures, and the systems within which health is protected and maintained. The database includes descriptions of ongoing projects and completed publications from health technology assessment organizations.

7. *NHS Economic Evaluation Database.* This database contains abstracts of articles describing economic evaluations of healthcare interventions, including:

- Cost-benefit analysis, which measures both costs and benefits in monetary values and calculates net monetary gains or losses (presented as a cost-benefit ratio)
- Cost-effectiveness analysis, which compares interventions with a common outcome (such as blood pressure level) to discover which produces the maximum outcome for the same input of resources in a given population
- Cost-utility analysis, which measures the benefits of alternative treatments or types of care by using clearly defined utility measures (such as quality-adjusted life years)

## Using Tertiary Source Materials

In reading an article that reviews other scientific papers or studies, results of a meta-analysis, practice guidelines, or material from the Cochrane Library, pay special attention to the list of papers in the references section. These references may be useful as you search for primary source articles.

Given the systematic effort and expertise that go into creating many of these tertiary source materials, you may now be wondering why you should do your own review of the literature. Why not simply use the excellent output of others on the topic of your choice? The answer is threefold:

1. The purpose of your review of the literature may not be exactly what has been included in these tertiary source materials.
2. A secondary or tertiary source document will inevitably contain a bias that you may or may not recognize. So far as that goes, your review of the primary source materials will also contain a bias. The advantage of doing your own review is that of experience—you know what the researchers said they did and how you interpreted their methods and results. You do not have that level of understanding if you read someone else's synthesis or review of the same documents.
3. Finally, you will not truly own the literature without examining the actual, primary source documents yourself. This is especially important for future research. On the other hand, if your goal is to gain a better understanding about what interventions or treatments are effective, then using one or more of the tertiary source documents may be the most efficient strategy.

Each of the four examples of tertiary source information has strengths and weaknesses. Reviews can vary in thoroughness and quality. There are no standards for review articles, as has been pointed out by others in the field. The same concern applies to a meta-analysis. A statistical methodology does not automatically confer objectivity. How the studies were selected initially, the quality of those original studies, and the appropriateness of the meta-analytic techniques are important considerations. Practice guidelines were developed for practitioners, and the quality of the research and ways in which the studies were combined to arrive at the guidelines may vary. Finally, the emphasis in the systematic reviews by the Cochrane Collaborative is on randomized trials. There is a vast amount of useful information from research studies that do not use that particular methodological design, and those studies are not emphasized in the Cochrane Library. In summary, you should seriously consider using tertiary source documents, but only as an adjunct to primary and secondary source materials.

## The Web: Beware of Readily Available Resources

The World Wide Web (www), which is currently the most popular system for accessing the Internet, offers expanding opportunities for the reviewer of the literature. One of the first places to explore is the NLM at http://www.nlm.gov. The NLM, which is part of the National Institutes of Health (NIH), has developed and maintains MEDLINE and other health-related databases. The website of the NIH is http://www.nih.gov. Both of these sites—NLM and NIH—can also be found by typing in these names in most search engines.

Other sites to explore include professional associations that publish journals, for example, the American Medical Association, which publishes *JAMA*, or the American Sociological Society, which publishes the *Journal of Health and Social Behavior*. Alternatively, you could search for the names of specific journals, such as the *American Journal of Public Health or Science*. Appendix A includes a list of some of the more well-known scientific associations and their websites.

## Nonfederal Web-Based Citation Indexes

Web-based citation indexes that are not part of the federal government (such as MEDLINE or CINAHL) have emerged since approximately

2004. These newcomers fall into two broad categories: those that are free and those that require an institutional or individual subscription.

Examples of the freely accessible indexes include Google Scholar (by the Google search engine), Scirus (by Elsevier, largest publisher of medical and scientific publications), CiteSeerX (by academics and researchers with a focus on computer and information science), and GetCITED (an online, member-controlled database of academic publications and citations of journal articles and book chapters).

Other citation indexes require a subscription and are usually available through libraries, especially university-based libraries. Examples include Scopus (by Elsevier, the publisher) and Thomson ISI's Web of Science, which includes the Science Citation Index (described in the next section). Check with the librarian at your university or your public library to see if it has a subscription to one of these indexes and determine whether or not you can gain free access to them.

In reviewing the literature, the logical question to ask is, "Should I use one of these other non-NLM indexes instead of (or in addition to) one of the other more well-established indexes such as MEDLINE (or PubMed)?" The answer is still in debate. You might explore one of these, such as Google Scholar, to see for yourself how the results of a limited search compare to those of the same search through PubMed.

## Citation Index: A Useful Tool Once You Know What You Want

After you are well into the process of locating specific journals and doing an initial reading of primary source materials, determine whether there are some individuals who consistently have been associated with the topic of interest. For example, are there key scientists who were the first to do this kind of research or authors whose seminal papers are almost always cited by others in their publications? If so, consider using the Science Citation Index (or its social sciences counterpart, the Social Science Citation Index) to identify other scientific publications in which the researchers list the papers by the key authors. Citation indexes are available in print (and electronic) form in most research libraries; the reference librarian will be able to help you locate and use such indexes.

In one sense, these citation indexes work backwards. For example, suppose that two fictitious researchers, Smith and Jones, published the first major study of quality of life of women with breast cancer in 1956 in the fictitious *Journal of American Health,* and their research was so important that most other researchers in the future cited that original paper. Now, years later, you want to identify all studies on this topic that have been reported since the Smith and Jones 1956 paper. Using the Science Citation Index, you look up Smith and Jones, and among their many publications, you locate the 1956 *Journal of American Health* article. Listed under that article will be a list of other studies, from 1956 to the present, that included the Smith and Jones article in the reference lists of their papers. In other words, the Smith and Jones 1956 paper was cited by these other authors. Such a list could be invaluable in a review of the literature because it quickly and efficiently gives you a list of potentially related articles that you can then examine and consider including in your review of the literature.

## Others Kinds of Resources: Recent Developments

There are two other sources of literature related to the health sciences literature that may become useful over time. They are described here not as a recommendation, but more as a suggestion that you keep an eye on them; check them out over the next few years, and decide for yourself whether either might be useful to you as you review the scientific literature.

### Grey Literature

This source consists of publications such as papers presented at scientific meetings, preliminary reports, technical reports, or government reports or documents. What makes this literature grey is that it is not produced by commercial publishers and is often very difficult to obtain. The term grey literature was described in a nongrey journal in 1990.[15] A professional conference meets periodically, and there is an effort to increase the acquisition and availability of grey literature about public health and health policy in libraries.[16] The website for further information is sponsored by the New York Academy of Medicine and is located at http://www.nyam.org/library/pages/grey_literature_report.

*Wikipedia*

Wikipedia is a free encyclopedia written and edited by the public. It was initially made available on the Web in 2001 and includes a broad range of topics that go beyond health-related information. It is not peer reviewed in the traditional sense of scientific journals, but it is a source that is increasingly being used by the public. Wikipedia can be accessed on the Web at http://en.wikipedia.org.

# TIPS ON SEARCHING FOR SOURCE DOCUMENTS

## Snowballing Technique: Developing Ownership of the Literature

Use what is known as the snowball technique to find more references. A snowball gathers snow as it rolls down the hill, and by the same token, your goal should be to use references in the papers or books you have read to gather more references. Even if a particular article in a journal is not relevant to the topic under review, some of the references might be. Build a list of references until you begin to see the same references over and over again. In fact, an author's failure to cite an important article in a current publication might suggest that this author did not fully read the literature, which might also make you question the quality of the study. You will know that you are beginning to own the literature when you read a few sentences about a study cited by an author and you immediately think to yourself, "Oh yes, that was the study by Smith and Jones in which they found that . . ." even before you see the reference to Smith and Jones at the end of the description.

## Timeliness of the Science: A Comparison of Sources

One consideration in reviewing the literature might be whether to include the most recent findings on a topic. Unfortunately, by the time a scientific paper is published in a peer-reviewed journal, the results are already out of date in some fields. Probably the most current knowledge about a topic can be found in papers presented at scientific meetings— but this applies only to the day or week they are presented. The disadvantage of presentations at scientific meetings is that they usually have not been subjected to the rigorous review process required of papers published in peer-reviewed journals. Materials made available on the Internet might also be very recent, but they are probably even more suspect if they have not gone through the peer-review process. The exception might be online, full-text papers in peer-reviewed journals available on the Internet. Examples of online journals are included in Appendix A. In general, the most recent published studies are papers in scientific journals, followed by those described in the annual reviews, followed finally by books.

If you restrict the review to scientific, peer-reviewed, hard-copy, published journals, then how recent is recent? The time from completion of a study (or the end of the study period, because it is not always clear when the study actually ended) to publication varies from study to study and field to field. Try to get a sense of a relative definition of recentness for papers in some journals by noting when the papers were submitted or accepted and when they were published. You will need to delve further, however, to discover how much time elapsed between the completion of the study and when the paper was submitted or accepted.

Take, for example, all of the patient-related articles that were original contributions published in the June 1998 issue of *JAMA*. There were 14 such articles, summarized in Exhibit 3-3, of which two did not provide information about when the data were collected or the study period ended. As shown in the last column of Exhibit 3-3, the range of time elapsed between the end of the data collection period (or end of study), and the publication of these 12 papers was 15 to 89 months. Thus, the information in the (then) latest issue of one of the foremost clinical journals in the world was published 3.67 years on average after the data were collected.

Research takes time, and good research often takes a lot of time. In thinking about the number of months or years elapsed between the end of study and publication of results, perhaps the most important issue to consider is how recent the findings have to be for the information to be meaningful to health providers and of benefit to their patients.

| Exhibit | |
|---|---|
| 3–3 | Time Elapsed between End of Study and Publication of Final Results in the June 1998 Issue of the *Journal of the American Medical Association* (*JAMA*) |

| Study Description | Date of Publication in JAMA | End of Study Period or Completion of Data Collection* | Number of Months Elapsed: End of Study to Publication |
|---|---|---|---|
| Socioeconomic Factors, Health Behaviors, and Mortality[17] | 6/3/98 | 3/1/94 | 50 |
| Perceived Prognosis and Treatment Preference[18] | 6/3/98 | 1/1/94 | 52 |
| Cigarette Smoking and Hearing Loss[19] | 6/3/98 | 1995 | 29 |
| Depressive Symptoms and Physical Decline[20] | 6/3/98 | 1992 | 65 |
| Death After Hospital Discharge[21] | 6/3/98 | 1994 | 41 |
| Low Back Pain in Industry[22] | 6/10/98 | N/A | N/A |
| Unintentional Cocaine Overdose[23] | 6/10/98 | 12/31/95 | 29 |
| Culture, Race, and Breast Cancer Stage[24] | 6/10/98 | N/A | N/A |
| Pain Management in Elderly Patients with Cancer[25] | 6/17/98 | 1995 | 17 |

*(continues)*

| Exhibit | | | | |
| --- | --- | --- | --- | --- |
| **3-3** | **Continued** | | | |

| Study Description | Date of Publication in JAMA | End of Study Period or Completion of Data Collection* | Number of Months Elapsed: End of Study to Publication |
| --- | --- | --- | --- |
| HIV Incidence among Young Adults[26] | 6/17/98 | 1993 | 53 |
| Risk Factors in Ischemic Heart Disease[27] | 6/24/98 | 1990 | 89 |
| Zinc Gluconate Lozenges for the Common Cold[28] | 6/24/98 | 3/97 | 15 |
| Adjusting Cesarean Delivery Rates[29] | 6/24/98 | 6/95 | 36 |
| Gastrostomies in Medicare Beneficiaries[30] | 6/24/98 | 12/93 | 53 |

*When only the year of data collection was reported, the ending date was set to December of that year, unless otherwise noted in the paper. N/A = Not Available.

# Caroline's Quest: Managing the Search

For her thesis research, Caroline was interested in studying the characteristics of teenage girls who smoke. She was especially interested in exploring whether there was a link between smoking and depression. In order to design her study, Caroline first needed to know what the research literature had shown about both the prevalence of smoking in that age and gender group and what kinds of characteristics had been studied thus far. She knew from previous reading that race or ethnic origin, socioeconomic status, and rural/urban location were probably important factors, but she was not sure what other kinds of characteristics had been studied.

After talking with Professor Dickerson, Caroline decided to begin by briefly reading pertinent chapters in a few reference books, then concentrating her search for primary source documents by looking in MEDLINE, and next examining some tertiary source documents beginning with the Cochrane Library.

At the library, Caroline skimmed the material on the topic of smoking and teenagers in the reference books and made some notes about these reference materials under key sources in the Paper Trail folder, as shown in Exhibit 3-4.

Before doing a MEDLINE search, Caroline listed some key words and set some initial restrictions for the search. She decided to focus only on American teenagers, with an age range of 13–18 years, if possible. She also wanted to limit her MEDLINE search to the most recent 10 years. Due to Professor Dickerson's guidance, she was aware that the definitions and terms for her search could be modified as she learned more about her topic.

Caroline wrote this information in the notes document in her Paper Trail folder in order to have a record of her decisions about the MEDLINE search. Her notes are shown in Exhibit 3-5.

| Exhibit | |
| --- | --- |
| **3-4** | **Key Sources Page in the Paper Trail Folder in Caroline's Lit Review Master Folder** |

Centers for Disease Control and Prevention. *Preventing tobacco use among young people: A report of the surgeon general: At a glance.* Atlanta, GA: National Center for Chronic Disease Prevention and Health Program; 1994.

| Exhibit | |
|---------|---|
| **3-5** | **Notes Page in the Paper Trail Folder in Caroline's Lit Review Master Folder** |

**Subject characteristics**
- Teenage—ages 13–18 years
- Smoking—use cigarette smoking only

**Prevalence**—be sure to get prevalence (rate of people currently smoking divided by total number at risk for smoking). May need to do this on a year-by-year basis. Wonder if I can get this for the entire age period? May want to set up a graph showing prevalence by year for each age.

**Limit search to the following:**
- The most recent 10 years, at least initially
- Focus only on American teenagers because they might differ from other cultures
- Separate different ethnic groups within the United States, e.g., Caucasian, African American, Asian, American Indian—there may be different characteristics associated with smoking within each ethnic group
- Limit search to English language journals only
- Check review articles, then go to the actual studies

Next she turned to the page titled "key words" in the Paper Trail folder and described the purpose of her literature review and some of the key words that she would use initially. Exhibit 3-6 is a record of what she wrote.

Caroline was able to access a variety of electronic bibliographic databases, such as MEDLINE, from the computer in her office, rather than go to the library. She also had two options for accessing the MEDLINE database. One was through PubMed, which was free via the Internet, and the other was through the OVID system, which was available through the biomedical library she used. Caroline felt fortunate because Professor Dickerson had told her that not all university libraries provide OVID free of charge to its users. Each access method had slightly different capabilities, although both provided a gateway to MEDLINE. She decided to use the PubMed system initially.

| Exhibit | |
| --- | --- |
| **3-6** | **Key Words Page in the Paper Trail Folder in Caroline's Lit Review Master Folder** |

**Purpose**
What are the characteristics of teenage girls who smoke during the period 1985 to the present in the United States?
**Key Words**
  smoking
  cigarettes
  teenage girls
  prevalence of smoking among teenage girls

Caroline logged onto the Internet, and before going to the PubMed website, she checked the home page of the NLM (www.nlm.nih.gov) to see whether any new features had become available. Then she went directly to the PubMed site to begin her MEDLINE search. The PubMed screen she went to first is shown in Figure 3-1.

Using the PubMed search capability, Caroline began her search with the key word phrase *smoking/epidemiology* and then restricted the search by the age and nationality criteria she had previously established. A copy of Caroline's first query, which retrieved 12,132 documents, is shown in Figure 3-2.

Caroline applied the search restrictions she had decided on earlier and recorded the results in the notes subsection of her paper trail. Her search resulted in 2,198 references, as shown in Exhibit 3-7.

Next, Caroline rapidly scanned the titles and abstracts of each of the 2,198 citations until she found a title relating to adolescents and smoking: the 2006 Harris et al. citation shown in Figure 3-3.

She examined the abstract, shown in Figure 3-4. Then she returned to the citations list and clicked on See Related Articles to find additional studies on the same topics.

## Figure 3-1

PubMed website that Caroline accessed to use MEDLINE. *Source:* Copyright Netscape Communications Corporation, 2006. All rights reserved. Netscape, Netscape Navigator, and the Netscape logo are registered trademarks of Netscape in the United States and other countries. PubMed is in the public domain; their availability is appreciated.

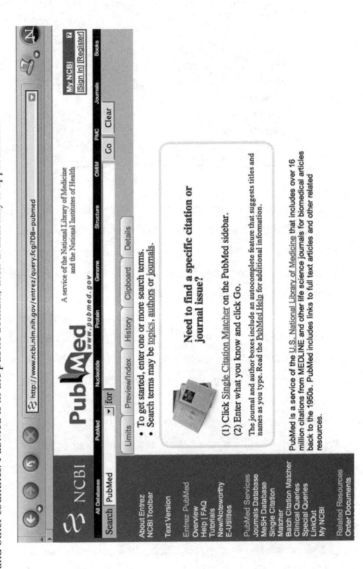

## Figure 3-2

Results of Caroline's initial query of the MEDLINE database using "smoking/epidemiology" as the key word phrase. *Source: Adapted from PubMed, the National Library of Medicine. Adapted with permission from Netscape Communications Corporation, 2006. All rights reserved. Netscape, Netscape Navigator, and the Netscape logo are registered trademarks of Netscape in the United States and other countries.*

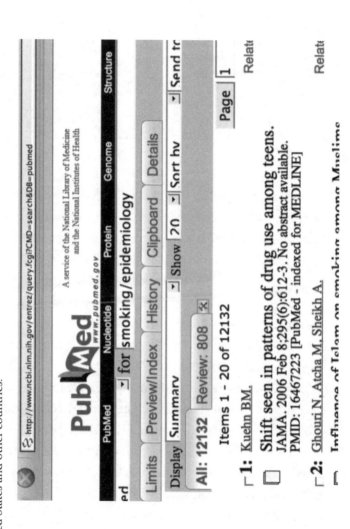

| Exhibit | |
| --- | --- |
| **3-7** | **Notes Page in the Paper Trail Folder in Caroline's Lit Review Master Folder** |

| Key words | Number of references |
| --- | --- |
| smoking/epidemiology | 12,132 |
| English language | 10,646 |
| human subjects | 10,615 |
| adolescents | 3,770 |
| females | 3,179 |
| 1966–2006 | 2,198 |

Caroline also explored some of the other electronic bibliographic databases such as CancerLit and CINAHL. Much of what she had found in MEDLINE was included in those two databases, although there were a few differences. Then she downloaded the papers she needed for those that were available electronically. For those that weren't, she made a trip to the biomedical library and made a photocopy of each of the papers. She knew that if the journals were not available online or in the library, then she could talk to the reference librarian about getting a copy of what she needed through Inter Library Loan.

Later, Caroline returned to the Web to look for reviews in the Cochrane Collaboration. She reasoned that these tertiary source materials might provide additional references of original research studies. She logged onto the Cochrane Collaboration home page at http://www.cochrane.org.

She clicked the Review Abstracts link on the home page in order to determine whether any Cochrane reviews had been completed for smoking and found a list of reviews to date at the next site.

Caroline decided to examine some other tertiary sources. She was particularly interested in looking in the *Annual Review of Public Health* to see whether there was an article on her topic. She reasoned that a current review would give her a list of up-to-date references of original studies that

**Figure 3-3**

Example of reference from MEDLINE. *Source:* Adapted from PubMed, the National Library of Medicine, 2006. PubMed is a free resource that is developed and maintained by the National Center for Biotechnology Information (NCBI), at the U.S. National Library of Medicine (NLM), located at the National Institutes of Health (NIH).

☑ **3:** Harris KM, Gordon-Larsen P, Chantala K, Udry JR.    Related Articles, Links

▣  **Longitudinal trends in race/ethnic disparities in leading health indicators from adolescence to young adulthood.**
Arch Pediatr Adolesc Med. 2006 Jan;160(1):74-81.
PMID: 16389215 [PubMed - indexed for MEDLINE]

# Figure 3-4

Abstract Caroline chose to examine. *Source:* Adapted from PubMed, the National Library of Medicine. Permission granted by the American Medical Association, 2006. All rights reserved. Harris KM, Gordon-Larsen P, Chantala K, Udry JR. Longitudinal trends in race/ethnic disparities in leading health indicators from adolescence to young adulthood. Arch Pediatr Adolesc Med. 2006 Jan; 160(1):74–81.

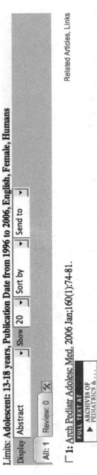

Limits: **Adolescent: 13-18 years, Publication Date from 1996 to 2006, English, Female, Humans**

Display  Abstract    Show  20    Sort by    Send to

All: 1    Review: 0

Related Articles, Links

☐ **1:** Arch Pediatr Adolesc Med. 2006 Jan;160(1):74-81.

FULL TEXT AT
▲ ARCHIVES OF
    PEDIATRICS & . . . .

**Longitudinal trends in race/ethnic disparities in leading health indicators from adolescence to young adulthood.**

Harris KM, Gordon-Larsen P, Chantala K, Udry JR.

Carolina Population Center, Schools of Public Health and Medicine, The University of North Carolina at Chapel Hill, University Square, 123 West Franklin Street, Chapel Hill, NC 27516-3997, USA.

OBJECTIVE: To use ethnically diverse, national data to examine longitudinal trends in race/ethnic disparities in 20 leading health indicators from Healthy People 2010 across multiple domains from adolescence to young adulthood. Much of what is known about health disparities is based on cross-sectional measures collected at a single time point. DESIGN, SETTING, AND PARTICIPANTS: Nationally representative data for more than 14 000 adolescents enrolled in wave I (1994-1995) or wave II (1996) of the National Longitudinal Study of Adolescent Health (Add Health) and followed up into adulthood (wave III; 2001-2002). We fit longitudinal regression models to assess and contrast the trend in health indicators among racial/ethnic groups of adolescents as they transition into adulthood. MAIN OUTCOME MEASURES: Diet, inactivity, obesity, tobacco use, substance use, binge drinking, violence, sexually transmitted diseases, mental health, and health care access. RESULTS: Diet, inactivity, obesity, health care access, substance use, and reproductive health worsened with age. Perceived health, mental health, and exposure to violence improved with age. On most health indicators, white and Asian subjects were at lowest and Native American subjects at highest risk. Although white subjects had more favorable health in adolescence, they experienced greatest declines by young adulthood. No single race/ethnic group consistently leads or falters in health across all indicators. CONCLUSIONS: Longitudinal data indicate that, for 15 of 20 indicators, health risk increased and access to health care decreased from the teen and adult years for would be useful to examine. She went first to the annual reviews website (http://www.annualreviews.org) and then to the site for the *Annual Review of Public Health* (http://publhealth.annualreviews.org). She did not find any review articles that were specific to her topic; therefore, she decided to concentrate on reading the papers she had either downloaded or photocopied to decide which of those should be included in her review. Then she would use the references from those papers to help her identify additional studies. Perhaps later she would consider using the Science Citation Index.

## REFERENCES

1. Poikolainen K. Alcohol and mortality: A review. *J Clin Epidemiol*. 1995;48:455–456.
2. Hunt DL, McKibbon KA. Locating and appraising systematic reviews. *Ann Intern Med*. 1997;126:532–538.
3. Weed DL. Methodologic guidelines for review papers. *J Natl Cancer Inst*. 1997; 89:6–7.
4. Oxman AD, Guyatt GH, Cook DJ, Jaeschke R, Heddle N, Keller J. An index of scientific quality for health reports in the lay press. *J Clin Epidemiol*. 1993;46: 987–1001.
5. Oxman AD. Checklists for review articles. *Br Med J*. 1994;309:648–651.
6. Breslow RA, Ross SA, Weed DL. Quality of reviews in epidemiology. *Am J Public Health*. 1998;88:475–477.
7. Fagard RH, Staessen JA, Thijs L. Advantages and disadvantages of the meta-analysis approach. *J Hypertens Suppl*. 1996;14:S9–S12; discussion S13.
8. Egger M, Smith GD. Meta-analysis. Potentials and promise. *Br Med J*. 1997; 315:1371–1374.
9. Egger M, Smith GD, Phillips AN. Meta-analysis: Principles and procedures. *Br Med J*. 1997;315:1533–1537.
10. Davey Smith G, Egger M, Phillips AN. Meta-analysis. Beyond the grand mean? *Br Med J*. 1997;315:1610–1614.
11. Egger M, Smith GD. Bias in location and selection of studies. *Br Med J*. 1998; 316:61–66.
12. Egger M, Schneider M, Smith GD. Meta-analysis—spurious precision—meta-analysis of observational studies. *Br Med J*. 1998;316:140–144.
13. Davey Smith G, Egger M. Meta-analysis: Unresolved issues and future developments. *Br Med J*. 1998;316:221–225.

14. Field MJ, Lohr KN. *Guidelines for Clinical Practice: From Development to Use*. Washington, DC: Committee on Clinical Practice Guidelines, Division of Health Care Services, Institute of Medicine; 1992.

15. Alberani V, Pietrangeli P, Mazza A. The use of grey literature in health sciences: A preliminary survey. *Bull Med Libr Assoc*. 1990;78(4):358–363.

16. Gray B. Sources used in health policy research and implications for information retrieval systems. *J Urban Health*. 1998;75(4):842–852.

17. Lantz PM, House JS, Lepkowski JM, Williams DR, Mero RP, Chen J. Socioeconomic factors, health behaviors, and mortality: Results from a nationally representative prospective study of US adults. *JAMA*. 1998;279:1703–1708.

18. Weeks JC, Cook EF, O'Day SJ, et al. Relationship between cancer patients' predictions of prognosis and their treatment preferences. *JAMA*. 1998;279: 1709–1714.

19. Cruickshanks KJ, Klein R, Klein BE, Wiley TL, Nordahl DM, Tweed TS. Cigarette smoking and hearing loss: The epidemiology of hearing loss study. *JAMA*. 1998;279:1715–1726.

20. Penninx BWJH, Guralnik JM, Ferrucci L, Simonsick EM, Deeg DJH, Wallace RB. Depressive symptoms and physical decline in community-dwelling older persons. *JAMA*. 1998;279:1720–1726.

21. Mullins RJ, Mann NC, Hedges JR, et al. Adequacy of hospital discharge status as a measure of outcome among injured patients. *JAMA*. 1998;279:1227–1231.

22. van Poppel NMN, Koes BW, van der Ploeg T, Smid T, Bouter LM. Lumbar supports and education for the prevention of low back pain in industry: A randomized controlled trial. *JAMA*. 1998;279:1789–1794.

23. Marzuk PM, Tardiff K, Leon AC, et al. Ambient temperature and mortality from unintentional cocaine overdose. *JAMA*. 1998;279:1795–1800.

24. Lannin DR, Mathews HF, Mitchell J, Swanson MS, Swanson FH, Edwards MS. Influence of socioeconomic and cultural factors on racial differences in late-stage presentation of breast cancer. *JAMA*. 1998;279:1801–1807.

25. Bernabei R, Gambassi G, Lapane K, et al. Management of pain in elderly patients with cancer. *JAMA*. 1998;279:1877–1882.

26. Rosenberg PS, Biggar RJ. Trends in HIV incidence among young adults in the United States. *JAMA*. 1998;279:1894–1899.

27. Lamarche B, Tchernof A, Mauriege P, et al. Fasting insulin and apolipoprotein B levels and low-density lipoprotein particle size as risk factors for ischemic heart disease. *JAMA*. 1998;279:1955–1961.

28. Macknin ML, Piedmonte M, Calendine C, Janosky J, Wald E. Zinc gluconate lozenges for treating the common cold in children: a randomized controlled trial. *JAMA*. 1998;279:1962–1967.

29. Aron DC, Harper DL, Shepardson LB, Rosenthal GE. Impact of risk-adjusting cesarean delivery rates when reporting hospital performance. *JAMA*. 1998;279: 1968–1972.

30. Grant MD, Rudberg MA, Brody JA. Gastrostomy placement and mortality among hospitalized Medicare beneficiaries. *JAMA*. 1998;279:1973–1976.

# 4

# Documents Folder: How to Select and Organize Documents for Review

This chapter is about how to select, organize, and keep track of all of the documents you use in a review of the literature. It includes the following sections:

- How to Select the Documents for Your Review
- What Is a Documents Folder?
- How to Organize a Documents Folder
- How to Remember Where You Put the Documents
- Caroline's Quest: Assembling a Documents Folder

# HOW TO SELECT THE DOCUMENTS FOR YOUR REVIEW

Selecting documents to include as possible candidates for your literature review is your next task. Reviewing the abstract, skimming the document, and downloading or photocopying the document are the three steps of the Matrix Method process for selecting documents.

## Review the Abstract

If the document is an original research article, then quickly read the abstract to see whether it is relevant to your topic. This strategy is most efficient if the abstract is available online in a database such as MEDLINE. Unfortunately, not all papers have an abstract, nor do the electronic bibliographic databases provide abstracts for some kinds of documents. For example, editorials usually do not include an abstract, yet such a document may include an important issue or a significant reference. Furthermore, some journals do not require an abstract for any of the papers. For documents with those limitations, go to the actual journal or source to determine whether they need to be considered for your review.

## Skim the Document

If either the title of the article or the abstract appears to be relevant to your topic or the study has been mentioned in a secondary or tertiary source document, the next step is to examine the original article briefly. It is more efficient if you can find the article as a full-text, online document—in other words, reprinted in its entirety in electronic form. Sometimes you will not be so fortunate, nor should you limit your search to only those articles available in electronic form. This is usually not a complete set of articles, and the sample of such journals might be biased.

After you have access to the paper, skim it briefly to determine whether it is relevant to your topic. Look not only at the abstract, but also the entire article, including the authors' statement of the purpose, the methods section, and the results. Consider the possibility that although the topic of a paper may be too specific for your review, the methods or the conclusions might have some relevance to a discussion in your final synthesis of the literature. If that is the case, download the article to your computer and store it in the Documents folder; this is discussed further in the next section.

This article selection process alone is just the beginning of your review of the literature; it is not sufficient for a review of the literature. Specifically, this stage involves only making a decision about whether to obtain a copy of the document for possible inclusion in your review.

## Get a Copy of the Document

Download electronic copies of relevant articles. If you have selected too many documents, then create a continuum for yourself from clearly essential to maybe relevant to remotely interesting, and download from the top of the continuum down until you run out of resources such as space or time. This means, however, that you may have to return to the source at an inconvenient time to reexamine one or more of the relevant articles. Make sure you record a copy of the URL where these papers are located in your Paper Trail folder.

If you want to include a document that is not in electronic form, you need to talk to a reference librarian about obtaining permission to make one copy for your use. It is important to abide by rules regarding copyright permission in making such a copy. Once a copy is available, you can scan it and store it in your Documents folder.

After you have selected a set of source documents, the next step is to use them to further expand the Documents folder in your Lit Review master folder.

# WHAT IS A DOCUMENTS FOLDER?

The Documents folder in the Lit Review master folder consists of one copy of each of the papers or source documents assembled for the literature review. In the years before photocopy machines or download capabilities were routinely available, you would have written to the author and asked for a reprint of the paper. Until recently, most scientific journals offered authors these reprints free or at cost. The practice of requesting a reprint is not as common now as in the past because most journals are available in major research libraries, through interlibrary loan, or more recently as full-text files on the Internet, and users can simply make a copy themselves. The term *reprint* is still with us, however, and occasionally you hear a collection of journal articles assembled for a review of the literature referred to as a "reprint file." Thus, the Documents folder is the same as a reprint file.

Think of the Documents folder as your database of source documents. Your database will be incomplete, however, because some documents are too large (such as books), unavailable (the journal is not available electronically), or restricted (such as proprietary materials owned by a private company). Maintain a list of all source documents that are important for your review, whether or not a copy is available. Often books can be obtained through interlibrary loan, and a copy of an article in an unavailable journal might be requested through the same source or from the author. Proprietary materials present another problem that may not be surmounted, but listing those that appear to be relevant in an appendix in your synthesis will indicate the thoroughness of your search. Bear in mind that proprietary documents are not usually included in the final review of the literature. However, for completeness in your list of source documents, you should record a citation of such a document in case you eventually find a source that is publicly available. An example might be a formerly classified report that has been declassified.

## Advantages of a Documents Folder

The advantage of maintaining a documents folder is being able to find your copy of a document when you need it. Even experienced researchers sometimes have trouble locating their copies of source documents. Occasionally, these seasoned veterans take the precaution of making multiple copies and spreading them around in several files in order to increase the likelihood of finding a copy when they need it. A documents folder in a lit review master folder solves that problem by providing a reservoir for research articles they have used in a review of the literature.

## HOW TO ORGANIZE A DOCUMENTS FOLDER

Just having a copy of a source document in the Documents folder does not guarantee that you will be able to find it efficiently the next time you need it. To bring order to the Documents folder, organize the materials by year of publication.

Create a file for the documents you have selected chronologically from earliest to latest. As you accumulate a list of source documents, maintain this in chronological order. Any further organization of the articles in the Documents folder, such as alphabetizing or grouping together by content area within a year, probably is not necessary.

The goal of this chronological sequence is twofold: (1) to arrange the source documents in the Documents folder for use in the next step, that of constructing the review matrix, and (2) to provide a quick index for efficiently finding a particular source document at a later time. When you have reached the point of diminishing returns by apparently exhausting all of the references that can be added, and you have organized the Documents folder in chronological order, you are ready to advance to the next step, that of constructing the review matrix. Bear in mind, however, that you probably will find more references and add more source materials to the Documents folder while constructing the review matrix and even later while writing a synthesis of the literature.

## HOW TO REMEMBER WHERE YOU PUT THE DOCUMENTS

Losing track of where you stored your reprints is an occupational hazard. Researchers, policy analysts, science writers, and other professionals in the health sciences who systematically and critically review the literature on multiple subjects face this problem. Regardless of the scope of the tasks or the setting, everyone experiences the same problem—how to find his or her materials, even when the information is stored in a lit review master folder. Some kind of tracking or indexing system is needed.

In this section, a simple tracking system is described that consists only of key words, references, and locations. A more sophisticated system, the Matrix Indexing System, is described in Chapter 8. The simple system, described here, will suffice to get you started.

Consider the following scenario: Your have three lit review master folders that contain pdf files of 30 or 40 research studies in each of the documents folders that you have assembled over considerable time; you cannot remember the details of all of the reprints or even the key words, and you often need to find a specific paper in a hurry because of a report or grant deadline, a paper you are preparing, or a request from someone for information. Furthermore, the hours spent trying to find a copy of a document takes time away from the task that you actually need to accomplish, such as completing the study or writing the report.

By the way, if you have more than one lit review master folder, then give them different labels. For example, one might be the Diabetes master folder, and the other might be the Maternal and Child Health master folder. If you always use the terms *master folder* or *lit review master*, then it is easier for you to use key words in a search for all the lit review folders on your desktop. Consistency in naming pays off! Likewise, when you create a documents folder within each of those master folders, then give it the same label as with the master folder, e.g., Diabetes Documents folder or Maternal and Child Health Documents folder. Labeling the folders with short names is best; this saves a lot of keyboarding.

The key to accessing your own store of information quickly and efficiently is to create a tracking system. Suppose that you have added new source documents to one of the documents folders over the past several years. How do you remember what is there? You need a system that lists the contents of each documents folder. As part of that index, you could indicate which documents were used in the initial review. You could also index notes and other materials in the paper trail, but for the sake of simplicity, only the tracking of the Documents folder is described here.

One of the simplest ways to index the source documents is to maintain a chronological list of source documents in the Documents folder. Consider using the table option in your word processor to create such a list, which includes the author(s), title, and year of publication. Store this table as a file in your Documents folder or on a central server that can be accessed by a group of people. Each time a reprint is added in the Documents folder, update the table.

A more sophisticated strategy for indexing the contents of an expanding documents folder is the Matrix Indexing System, which is described in Chapter 8. The simpler approach is this tracking system. Whichever system you use, the benefits accrue only if you keep the list up to date.

# Caroline's Quest: Assembling a Documents Folder

Caroline's next task was to choose which of the 15 research articles she would abstract in the review matrix. First she sorted the papers by year of publication and began with the oldest paper, published in 1992. She read the abstract and skimmed the entire paper, making a few notes about questions she would return to later when she abstracted the final set of papers. At this point, Caroline was not doing any abstracting. In fact, she had not even decided which topics she would use as the basis for abstracting the studies. As she read, however, she made notes of potential topics for the review matrix. Of the 15 papers she scanned, Caroline chose nine of the studies as possible candidates for abstracting in the review matrix on characteristics of adolescent girls who smoke.

"Well, that step was easy," Caroline commented to Professor Dickerson at their weekly meeting. She showed him the Lit Review master folder on her laptop with her notes in the Paper Trail folder and the copies of the nine articles in the Documents folder.

"What happened to the six papers you decided not to include?" Professor Dickerson asked her.

Caroline described how she chose only the most relevant ones.

Professor Dickerson understood her logic, but he cautioned, "You might want to leave the other six papers you found in your Documents folder even if you don't use them."

He paused at her quizzical look and added, "I've found that sometimes a study is referred to by an author and I wonder if I shouldn't consider it.

If I've deleted it from my Documents folder, then I have to go find it again. But if I just leave it in the folder, then I know I've read it and realized it wasn't useful. Since you've got a lot of storage space, think about the practice of including every paper you download."

Caroline made a note of this advice.

"Now, filing reprints is easy," Professor Dickerson continued. "But your job isn't done yet. You need to constantly be alert for more studies as you read each of these articles. If you find that there are some authors who are referenced frequently, then look them up in Science Citation Index to see whether you can find additional studies that also cited them." He grinned. "Use the snowball technique to find more studies," he advised.

"What if I haven't found all the right studies?" Caroline looked concerned. "I could be missing something that is a classic in the field and not even know it. Reviewing the literature seems like such a hit or miss kind of thing, even with the Matrix Method."

Professor Dickerson nodded, "I agree. You must constantly be looking for more studies. Abstracting the ones you have will probably help. You want to reach the point where you have the sense that you know who the researchers are and what research questions they have studied. In other words, you need to begin to own the literature."

"Okay, I understand how to use the documents. But what if all of the documents that I want to use have been gathered together already, say, in a special report on the Web? Do I have to make a copy of each one and put them in a documents folder in order to do a review of the literature?" Caroline was thinking about the effort it would take to find and download each of the papers—all in different journals, no doubt.

"No," Professor Dickerson responded. "If the documents are available elsewhere and convenient to use, then you do not have to download a copy. The Documents folder is meant to be a convenience for you and an organized way of maintaining a reprints file." He thought a minute and then continued, "Frankly, Caroline, I don't know of many situations in which all of the documents for a literature review have already been assembled in one place. You will also need to think about what to do with the articles themselves. One of the advantages of having a copy of an article when you abstract it for the review matrix is that you can mark it up as you read it. If possible, turn on track changes in your word processor and insert comments. You can highlight certain key parts or write questions to yourself on a sticky or create another blank document and write your questions and answers there. If you are working from an original in another database, then you can't mark it up."

He paused to let Caroline think about the pros and cons of downloading copies of the documents for her review, and then he continued, "Your task next week will be to read all of the articles and make some decisions about which column topics to use in your review matrix."

# 5

# Review Matrix: How to Abstract the Research Literature

This chapter describes how to set up a review matrix, choose topics for the matrix, and abstract each of the source documents based on these topics. The sections of this chapter are as follows:

- ⊙ What Is a Review Matrix?
- ⊙ How to Construct a Review Matrix
- ⊙ How to Arrange Documents for Use in a Review Matrix
- ⊙ How to Choose Column Topics for a Review Matrix
- ⊙ How to Abstract Documents in a Review Matrix
- ⊙ Fringe Benefits of the Abstracting Process
- ⊙ Caroline's Quest: Constructing a Review Matrix

# WHAT IS A REVIEW MATRIX?

A matrix is a box with rows and columns, like a spreadsheet. In a review matrix, the rows are for documents such as journal articles, and the columns are for the topics you will use to summarize each of those documents. A summary of an article in a review matrix describes only the most pertinent points about the topic. Table 5-1 shows a generic example in which the first two rows are journal articles and the columns are the first four topics of the review matrix.

For example, if you were interested in a review matrix summary of an article by the fictitious Professor Brown on his fictitious paper, *The Cure for the Common Cold*, the paper would be listed in the first row, and the topics you are going to use to describe that paper would be listed across the top of the review matrix. Professor Brown's archrival, Professor White, published a similar paper in 1989, which you also described. Table 5-2 illustrates how those two papers would look in the first part of a review matrix.

Thus, a review matrix is a rectangular arrangement, or a matrix, in which the rows always have the journal articles or papers listed down the left side, and the topics or issues that you are going to use to summarize each article are always listed across the top.

| Table | | | |
|-------|--|--|--|
| **5-1** | Generic Review Matrix | | |
| **Topic 1** *Example:* *Author, title, journal* | **Topic 2** *Example:* *Year* | **Topic 3** *Example:* *Purpose* | **Topic 4** *Example:* *Type of Study Design* |
| Journal article 1 | 1995 | Drug treatment for epilepsy | Experimental study |
| Journal article 2 | 1997 | Drug treatment for depression | Case-control study |

| Table | |
|---|---|
| **5–2** | **Review Matrix for Literature on Cure for the Common Cold** |

| Author, Title, Journal | Year | Purpose | Methodological Design |
|---|---|---|---|
| Brown, C.J. Cure for the common cold. *Journal of Scientific Wonder.* | 1987 | Compare drug X with a placebo for cold cure | Randomized clinical trial |
| White, R.M. A better cure for the common cold. *Journal of Better Science.* | 1989 | Compare drug Y with drug X for superior cold cure | Randomized clinical trial |

## Advantages of a Review Matrix

The reason for using the Matrix Method is to create order out of chaos. In a review of the literature, the chaos that you must deal with is too much information spread across too many journal articles or other source documents with too many details to remember. The order you are going to impose is that of organizing this information so that you can then think about it and use it efficiently. The review matrix provides a standard structure for creating order. Constructing a review matrix is like building a house. You will still need to furnish the house, in this case by reading and summarizing each article and putting that information in each cell, but the review matrix provides a place for everything, which allows you to concentrate efficiently and reliably on the information itself.

# HOW TO CONSTRUCT A REVIEW MATRIX

Constructing a review matrix as a basis for writing a synthesis in a literature review is a simple, three-step process:

1. *Organizing the documents.* Organize the Documents folder chronologically by arranging the source documents from the oldest to the most recent by year of publication.
2. *Choosing topics.* Set up the review matrix on your computer desktop using either the table function in a word processor or as a spreadsheet, and decide which topics to use for this review of the literature.
3. *Summarizing the documents.* Read and summarize each source document one at a time in chronological order, from oldest to most recent, and record your notes under each topic in the review matrix.

## HOW TO ARRANGE DOCUMENTS FOR USE IN A REVIEW MATRIX

Source documents should be organized chronologically, from the oldest to the most recent by year of publication. Most of the source documents that you will summarize in the review matrix probably will be research papers and other journal articles or book chapters. Most of the documents will be stored in the Documents folder in your Lit Review master folder, as discussed in Chapter 4.

## HOW TO CHOOSE COLUMN TOPICS FOR A REVIEW MATRIX

### What Is a Column Topic?

In a review of the literature, the three most important decisions you will make are (1) specifying the purpose of the literature review, (2) selecting the source documents, and (3) choosing the column topics. Column topics in a review matrix are the issues or concepts used to abstract each journal article or other source document.

For example, if one of the column topics is "sampling design," then your task in completing a review matrix is to identify the type of design used to select subjects for every study abstracted. If the authors did not describe the sampling design, then record its absence in that study by noting that it is not available (NA) or give your best guess, for example, "NA—probably volunteer subjects."

## Categories of Column Topics

Rarely will a review of the literature be so comprehensive as to include all of the column topics possible. When reviewing the scientific literature, consider two broad categories in thinking about the column topics you choose: (1) methodological characteristics of the study and (2) content-specific characteristics such as the theoretical or conceptual model, the types of results, or the implications for policy.

Most studies published in scientific journals in the health and behavior literature follow a standard format, as described in the section called "Anatomy of a Scientific Paper" in Chapter 2, and include a common set of methodological characteristics describing how the study was designed and analyzed. In choosing column topics, consider including some of these methodological characteristics. A list of methodological topics and a description of each are described in "Guidelines for a Methodological Review of the Literature" in Chapter 2.

Because these methodological topics will not be sufficient to describe a body of research, be sure to include topics that cover the content of the research. Choose topics based on their relevance to the purpose of your literature review.

## First Three Column Topics

Make it a practice to always let the first three columns in any review matrix be the same. Use these three columns to record fundamental information about each source document you abstract:

- Column 1: Author(s), title, name of journal
- Column 2: Year of publication
- Column 3: Purpose of the paper or source document

In the first column, record all of the names of multiple authors of a paper or book, not just the first three followed by et al. By including all authors, you will be in a better position to track all of the researchers involved in this kind of research. Look for the same researchers as authors of other papers later in time, whether or not they published together.

Setting aside a column for the year is important because that is the basis on which you will sort and index all source documents as well as the reprints in the Documents folder. Year of publication is the key to finding copies of articles quickly and efficiently.

The third column is used to describe the purpose of the document—why was the study done, or what was the purpose of the document? State the purpose in your own words. For a research study, try to describe the purpose as a research question. If you (or the authors of the paper) cannot describe the intended purpose in the form of a question, how can you (or they) know whether the question was answered? Describing the purpose may be difficult at times. Some authors do not provide a clear statement of purpose in the introduction section of a paper, and you may have to read the entire paper in order to determine what they intended to do.

The choice of the rest of the topics is up to you. This is a judgment call that will be based on the purpose of your literature review and your knowledge about the topic. Although there are no rules for generating a list of topics or choosing among them, what follows are some suggestions for a process that may be useful.

## Process for Choosing the Remaining Topics

What if you do not know what topics to choose other than the first three? Even if you are doing a literature review to find out something about the latest research in an unfamiliar field, you do know something about the topic. By the time you are ready to choose the column topics for a review matrix, you will have consulted reference books about the topic, read numerous abstracts on an electronic bibliographic database or in journals, and skimmed the papers of the source documents downloaded in the Documents folder. The four-step process to use in deciding which column topics to include is summarized here.

### Step 1—Read the Documents

Read all of the articles or source documents in the Documents folder in chronological order so that you can grasp the scope of the research.

This will also begin to give you a sense of how the research issues and methodologies have changed over time. For this second brief reading of the articles, the purpose is to gain enough of a perspective to choose column topics. Note that some of the documents may not be in electronic form. For example, you may have selected chapters in books or government reports. If possible, make a pdf file copy or order the reports. You can create a document in your Documents folder consisting of the citation for each of these nonelectronic materials and then refer to the hard copy when necessary.

## Step 2—List Important Issues

While reading the source documents, make a list of the most important issues, both methodological as well as content specific. For example, if some of the earlier studies used observational designs but later ones used experimental designs, then type of methodological design might be an important topic. Alternatively, if the area you are reviewing is limited to Medicare recipients, then under a subjects column, make a note of this selection criterion, but do not devote a column to a topic that will be the same for all studies.

## Step 3—Select Column Topics

After you have finished reading all of the source documents, select the topics that seem to be the most important from two standpoints: issues in the field and the purpose of your literature review. For example, suppose that you are reviewing the literature on worldwide epidemiology of HIV and are especially interested in the rates in South American countries compared with other parts of the world. With regard to content, you might set aside a column for how HIV status was assessed in each study. For purposes of your review, you might include another column for the country in which the subjects resided.

## Step 4—Add Column Topics

After you have begun to abstract the first few source documents, you may need to add some important topics. Plan for this addition in advance by reserving some blank columns in the review matrix. Additional topics can be added at any time. Be sure to go back and include the papers that you have already abstracted when you add those topics. Sometimes it is not possible to know the full range of topics until you have abstracted all of the documents. (If that happens, then the philosophy of the review matrix is working: the abstracting process enabled you to identify an important topic that you had not seen when you began.) Add the missing topics and abstract all of the papers again on that basis.

## A Matter of Thoroughness

At this point, you may be thinking that this amount of detail and effort requires too much commitment on your part, especially when your counterparts have already accomplished their review of the literature in a tenth of the time by simply using a search engine to locate a few studies and summarizing them.

Whether or not to proceed is fundamentally a decision that only you can make. Think about why you are doing a review of the literature and what the consequences will be of not doing it thoroughly. If you are trying to understand what is known about a specific subject or if you want to identify what is missing in a body of research, then you must own the literature. Can you take the chance that you have overlooked an important paper? Are you willing to design your own research study without knowing whether some other researcher already has addressed that very question? How thorough is thorough enough?

This also raises the question, "How many papers or source documents is enough? Is there a specific number to aim for?" The answer is "No." As you begin to read the source documents, ask yourself these questions:

- What is the time frame of this review? Do I examine research over the past five or ten years? Was there a seminal event such as the mapping of the human genome that marked a clear turning point in this research? Should I use that as the beginning of this time frame? You could go back ten years before this event and therefore increase the number of papers you select, but that might not be logical based on the purpose of the review.
- How specifically should the subject of this review be defined? For example, if the review is of outcomes of total knee replace-

ment surgery, was there a specific type of replacement part that you are interested in, thus that becomes part of the definition you are using? Perhaps there have only been seven papers published about this replacement part. You may want to broaden your definition. Alternatively, seven could be the total number of papers you include, and that number is sufficient.

There is no thoroughness index that will tell you when you have done enough. Your only guide to determining thoroughness is your own sense of knowing the literature well enough to own it. The Matrix Method is one way of approaching that type of ownership, but it is not a guarantee of thoroughness. If you decide to continue, the next step is to concentrate on a single article or paper at a time; read it thoroughly and abstract it based on the column topics. Then read and abstract the next source document until all have been examined.

# HOW TO ABSTRACT DOCUMENTS IN A REVIEW MATRIX

## Taking Notes

What do you do when you abstract an article? At the simplest level, you type a note about the topic in the area, or cell, where the row and column meet in the review matrix. By now, you have read each article at least twice, first to decide whether to download it to the Documents folder and second to make a decision about which column topics to use. Next comes the third and most intensive reading in which you will critically analyze the source documents—abstract each on the basis of the column topics, and in the process, construct the cells of the review matrix.

## Essential Tools

Never read an empirical paper without a calculator. Check the numbers and the percentages. Do the number of subjects in the tables of results add up to the numbers the researchers said they enrolled at the beginning of the study? All of this will help you understand what the authors did in conducting their study. Two other important tools to have at hand when critically reading a research paper are the highlighter tool in your word processor or spreadsheet for marking important sections of the paper and a sticky note or comment tool in your software for writing notes and questions on the paper itself.

## Recreate the Study in Your Mind

Be forewarned that simply recording information in the review matrix without reconstructing the study in your own mind does not constitute a critical review of the literature. In order to read a scientific paper thoroughly, you must essentially re-create the study by retracing the authors' steps. Begin by asking yourself questions such as what was their purpose, how did they go about doing the study, what were their results, and what was their logic in their interpretation of the results they found? In the process of understanding what the authors did, determine whether you agree scientifically with their purpose, methods, results, and interpretations. That is the critical part of critically reviewing the literature.

In one sense, each scientific paper is a story—a true story—and you have to recreate that story accurately in your own words in order to understand the paper fully. Make electronic notes in the margins of the paper as you read it. Highlight words that you do not understand or terms that the authors did not define and look them up. Highlight important parts of the paper such as the purpose or key results and draw diagrams of the time relationships. For example, when was the pretest administered? How much later was the intervention? How long did the intervention last, and how long after that was the posttest?

## Read in Chronologic Order

The chronologic order in which you read the papers is also important. Begin with the oldest paper, based on its publication date, and end with the most recent. The reason for reading in chronologic order is that the research of later papers should build on the results of a previous body of work. Perhaps the findings of one paper suggested a new theory for a future study, a new analytic method became available, or an old study was reanalyzed.

Of course the progress that you may see over time depends on the range of papers selected for your review, and there may be gaps in the progression of the science because of papers you overlooked or decided not to analyze. If this appears to be the case, you can always go back and include the missing articles.

## Write Notes in the Matrix

In constructing a review matrix, your task is to take each article or source material and record notes based on the column topics. The notes in the cells of the review matrix have to be concise and very short. Their purpose is to allow you to track the details of a study, not to summarize the entire article.

Occasionally, you will have included an article that is a review of other studies or a theoretical paper. In this case, you might want to ignore the column topics and make a note in the review matrix for that row about the importance of that paper or whether it is a good summary.

Other papers may include important points or quotes that you will want to remember without having to search back through all of the materials in the Documents folder. Write these more detailed notes in another document or on the computer equivalent of a sticky note and make a note in the matrix where further information was recorded.

An example of the process of reading a research paper in preparation for abstracting it in the review matrix is shown in Exhibit 5-1.

## Additional Information

In the meantime, as you read each source document, add to your list of references and photocopy or download additional articles that will be added to the Documents folder, as needed. Not everything will fit neatly under one of the column topics. If you are using a spreadsheet or word processor to create the review matrix, set aside a special section or file to include these notes. Remember to plan for expansion.

| Exhibit | |
|---|---|
| **5-1** | **How to Abstract a Research Paper** |

### INTRODUCTION SECTION

Begin with the introduction section of the paper. Rephrase the authors' purpose in your own words. Put it in the form of a research question. If the authors have not included a purpose—some do not—then state what you think their question is and make a note that they did not state the purpose.

### METHODS SECTION

Read and reread each part of the methods section of the paper until you have a clear idea of what the authors did. Sometimes authors (or editors) leave out important information. If so, describe what you think they did—but make a note that this was your opinion. In order to really understand the study, you need to re-create what the authors did in carrying it out. In other words, describe for yourself the procedures they used.

Now look at the numbers in the subsection about subjects and how they were selected for the study. Begin with the number of subjects—is it possible to trace how many were in the sample at the beginning of the study and how many subjects were lost as the study progressed? Subjects get lost for a variety of reasons; they might have died or moved away or simply may not have responded. This is where your calculator comes in. Figure out what the real response rate was; do not depend on the authors' calculations.

The reason this response rate is so important is that researchers run the risk of subject bias if the characteristics of the sample of subjects who end the study differ from those who began the study. For example, the authors may report that the response rate to a questionnaire was 87% (that is, 87% of the people who were asked to fill out the questionnaire actually did) or that the completion rate for an intervention was 45%. Anything less than 100% raises the possibility of a sample bias, but a rate alone does not indicate sample bias. The authors must compare the people who did and did not respond, and then describe in the paper what the differences were statistically. Many authors do not include that information. If they have not included it, then make a note of this potential weakness of the study.

Now take this same critical approach to reading about how the data were collected. Was a questionnaire or survey used? If so, what questions or items were included? Was research completed on the instrument itself before it was used in this study? For example, what do the authors report about the validity and reliability of the instrument? If data from a national study were used, then have the authors provided references so you can go back and get the information about how the data were collected? Do not automatically assume that a study was done correctly just because a national sample of subjects was drawn or this was part of a very large project. Read critically.

Continue to read each part of the methods section of the paper in this way. If you do not know what to look for, review the section called "Guidelines for a Methodological Review of the Literature" in Chapter 2.

### RESULTS SECTION

Reread the purpose of the paper, and then examine the results section to see whether the authors answered the research questions or hypotheses they initially stated. Were additional questions posed and answered in the process of addressing the main questions? Were there additional research questions that were not answered?

### DISCUSSION SECTION

As you read the paper, think about the strengths and weaknesses of the study, and then note whether the authors described the same problems or advantages. Note especially what additional research questions were not addressed. Ask yourself what the implications of the results were or the significance of these findings.

### REFERENCES

You might find it useful to make notes about the references at the end of each paper. Specifically, go through the references of each paper and add to your own list (in the Paper Trail folder) any that call for follow-up.

### ACKNOWLEDGMENTS

This column topic might be included in the review if issues such as funding source are relevant. For example, you might consider whether the funding source of a research project posed a potential conflict of interest, such as a study about the rates of teenage smoking that has been funded by the tobacco industry.

### REVIEWER-SPECIFIC TOPICS

A review matrix should be tailored to the purpose of your review of the literature. Rarely will a review be so comprehensive as to include all of the column topics

*(continues)*

| Exhibit | |
|---|---|
| **5-1** | **Continued** |

described previously here. In fact, you may choose to include only a few of the topics described previously and instead opt for some very specific topics of your own. For example, if your review of the literature is limited to experimental studies, then it might be redundant to have a column topic on experimental designs. Alternatively, if you believe that knowing which kinds of experimental designs would be important to understanding this literature, then you will need such a column topic. These reviewer-specific column topics may dominate the review of the literature, to the exclusion of many of the other topics listed.

### SOME GENERAL ADVICE

Rarely will you ever read straight through a paper in a linear fashion, from introduction to the discussion section. You may start out this way, but as you get into the paper, you will find it necessary to go back and recheck some of the details. For example, in the midst of the methods section you may jump ahead to the results section ("Did they really keep all of the subjects in the study who were enrolled at the beginning?") or in the middle of reading about the results, you may return to the Introduction section ("What did the authors say the purpose was?"). As you read these papers, keep a running dialogue with yourself about what the researchers intended to do, what they really did, what they reported they found, and what they actually found.

This double-checking is important. Do not assume anything, and do not give any author of a research paper the benefit of the doubt. In reviewing the literature, the best attitude is to be methodologically suspicious and ever doubtful.

# FRINGE BENEFITS OF THE ABSTRACTING PROCESS

## Overview

The reason for constructing a review matrix is to provide a basis for systematically analyzing the literature and writing a review of the literature in the form of a synthesis. Constructing a review matrix is both tedious and time consuming, but there are some additional advantages in the abstracting process itself, provided that you have done a thorough job of collecting the most relevant research papers on a subject. In the first place, you learn something about the sociology of the subject you are reviewing. Second, by taking apart and abstracting each study using the same set of topics, you are better able to state questions of your own. Finally, you begin to have a better sense of what is missing and areas in which new research is needed.

## Sociology of the Research Topic

As you carefully read and abstract each source document in chronological order, especially if they are research papers in a specific area, then you will begin to know the following:

- Who the researchers are and with whom they collaborate
- Where the research is being done
- Whether they tend to use the same data sets
- What the funding sources are
- Which studies are cited repeatedly

In other words, without consciously trying to, you begin to become aware of the sociology of this research topic as you abstract the studies.

### Who the Researchers Are

Knowing the names of the researchers is useful if you want to find related studies by running an author search on MEDLINE or one of the other electronic bibliographic databases. Science Citation Index is a useful source for finding other studies by authors not included in the group now familiar to you. Knowing who collaborates with whom is important when learning about a new research field. For example, what appears to be a widespread research effort being done by a multitude of different researchers may, on closer inspection, be the product of the same group or subgroup of collaborators who happen to be located in diverse university and nonacademic settings. There is nothing wrong with such an effort; in fact, it has become even more feasible with the advent of the Internet. Such information would be useful if you wanted to contact someone in that group and discovered that one of them was in your institution or a place nearby.

## Where the Research Is Done

In the process of abstracting, you will begin to notice where the authors are located geographically. Some research efforts take place in a single institution; others, as suggested previously, may be spread throughout the country. For example, most of the work in the area of evidence-based medicine was done at McMaster University, although there were some collaborators in other Canadian and American universities. If you were interested in pursuing that topic in greater depth, going to McMaster or contacting someone there might be the first place to start. Checking out the group's website for a list of current or prospective publications would also be useful.

## Data Sets They Have in Common

Often researchers in a related area use the same data set, such as one of the National Health Interview Surveys[1-3] or the National Health and Nutrition Examination Survey (NHANES). If you are familiar with how the data were gathered and what the strengths and limitations of these data sets are, then you are in a better position to evaluate the studies that used them. To locate studies based on these large-scale, nationally representative databases, use the database name, such as NHANES, as a key word search on MEDLINE.

## Funding Sources

If two or more studies have been funded by the same source, you might find research projects in the same area by looking up that funding source. For example, if a study has been funded by a research grant from the National Institute on Aging, then search on the National Institutes of Health database to see whether additional studies have been funded (see Chapter 3 for information about how to conduct an NIH RePORTER search). Some of the more recently funded studies still may be in progress, and the results will not have been published yet. It is also possible that some currently funded projects are being done by researchers other than those whose papers you have read, and they may be exploring different aspects of what is currently being published. In this case, consider contacting the principal investigators of these ongoing studies to find out something about their work. Whether you choose to take this extra step depends on why you are doing this review of the literature. Many private foundations also list research projects they have funded in the past or are currently funding. Look them up on the Internet.

### Same Basic References

When checking the references section at the end of most research papers published in health sciences journals, you may find that the same research papers are being cited repeatedly by the authors of the documents you are abstracting. If you have not included these papers in your own review, consider adding them to the list you are abstracting.

## Seeing What Is Missing

As you abstract each of the studies in your literature review, you are better able to develop your own questions about the research issues. Finding the answers to these questions will enable you to see the bigger picture. There is a real advantage for the person writing a grant proposal to see where the holes are in the current research on a topic. The abstracting process makes it possible for you to begin to see not only the issues that apparently have not been addressed but many of the methodological flaws as well. Discovering what is missing is part of owning the literature, and constructing the review matrix makes this possible.

# Caroline's Quest: Constructing a Review Matrix

After Caroline had arranged the reprints chronologically in the Documents folder in her Lit Review master folder, she was ready to choose the column topics for the review matrix. She reread each of the research papers quickly and jotted down further notes about which issues or topics appeared to be the most important. She also reviewed the list of methodological topics (as described in Chapter 2) that Professor Dickerson had

given her. She knew that she would not need all of the methodological topics, but some of them probably would be useful.

Caroline began by listing the first three topics that were standard in
every review matrix constructed using the Matrix Method: (1) authors, title,
and journal; (2) year of publication; and (3) purpose. Next, she decided to
concentrate on some of the methodological characteristics in her column
topics, and for that reason she chose the outcome variable, which she
recorded as the dependent variable in the review matrix. She knew that the
studies varied in their definition of smoking. Depending on the purpose of
each study, some authors concentrated only on cigarette smoking; others
included chewing tobacco.

The next column topic she wrote was independent variable. This was the
topic that would help her sort out which characteristics the authors had used
to look at variations in smoking behavior. Caroline continued to add topics, such as the number of subjects in the study and whether the study was
limited to females only or included both sexes.

Altogether, Caroline chose 17 topics, which she listed across the top of her
still blank review matrix. Eleven of those topics are shown in Exhibit 5-2,
which lists only the methodological topics plus a comment topic, which she
reserved for making notes about the strengths and weaknesses of each study.

Caroline left several columns blank so that she could add a few additional
topics as she abstracted the studies. She was ready to begin to abstract the
studies she had chosen.

Caroline began the abstracting process by setting aside the review matrix, taking out her calculator, and selecting the yellow highlighter on her
software, and turning to the first paper in the Documents folder. This was
the third time she had read this paper, but this was the most concentrated
reading. Caroline highlighted the sentence in the purpose section of the
paper and made a note of the dependent and independent variables. She
used her calculator to track the percentage of subjects who dropped out of
the study or who did not respond to the survey. Caroline continued to read
the paper thoroughly until she had a clear understanding of what the

| Exhibit | |
|---|---|
| **5–2** | Caroline's Review Matrix for Research Literature on Smoking by Adolescent Girls |

| Authors, Title, Journal | Year Pub | PURPOSE | VARIABLES | | SUBJECTS | | | | DATA | | COMMENTS |
|---|---|---|---|---|---|---|---|---|---|---|---|
| | | | Dependent | Independent | # of Subjects | Subject characteristics | Sample Design | Source or Instrument | Yr data collected | | |
| Wang, Fitzhugh, Westerfield, Eddy. Family & peer influences on smoking behavior among American adolescents: an age trend. *J Adoles Health.* | 1995 | What is influence of family and peers on adolescent smoking? | cigarette smoking only | peer by sex family—sibling, father, mother | 6,900 | male & female, 14–18 yrs | nat'l—random (82% response rate) | Nat'l Hlth Interv Surv | 1988–89 | • no response/non resp analysis for subjects<br>• no info on data collect instrument<br>• no race information |
| Altman, Levine, Coeytaux, Slade, Jaffe. Tobacco promotion and susceptibility to tobacco use among adol. aged 12–17 years in a nationally repres. sample. *AJPH.* | 1996 | What is relation between youth susceptibility to tobacco use and participation in promotional campaign? | suscep to tob.:<br>• non–tob. use<br>• suscep to tobac<br>• current tob. use<br>cigarette & chew tobacco | age, gender, tob. user in household, awareness of tob. promot, know friend owns promot item, particip in tob. promot, mail from tob., free sample | 1,047 | male & female, 12–17 yrs | nat'l—random (62% response rate) | author conduct sample—random digit dialing across U.S. | 1993 | • no resp/non-resp analysis<br>• no info on data collection instrument<br>• no race info |

*(continues)*

Exhibit 5-2 Continued

| Authors, Title, Journal | Year Pub | PURPOSE | VARIABLES | | SUBJECTS | | | DATA | | COMMENTS |
|---|---|---|---|---|---|---|---|---|---|---|
| | | | Dependent | Independent | # of Subjects | Subject characteristics | Sample Design | Source or Instrument | Yr data collected | |
| French & Perry. Smoking among adolescent girls; prevalence & etiology. *JAMWA*. | 1996 | To review lit on prevalence & etiology of smok by adolescent girls. | cigarette smoking | female, race | varies by study | female, 17–18 yrs | across multiple studies | varies | varies | Not an empirical study. Summary of literature only.<br>• info on race included. Note prevalence rates. |

purpose of the study was, how the authors had conducted the study, and what they had found.

Then Caroline turned to the review matrix and began to fill in the cells for that study under each of the column topics. After examining the list of references at the end of the paper, she added a few references to her list to look up in MEDLINE when she finished abstracting.

Caroline abstracted each paper immediately after reading it. Examples of three of the papers she abstracted, the Wang et al. study,[4] the Altman et al. paper,[5] and the French and Perry article[6] are shown in Exhibit 5-2. Although the paper by French and Perry was not an actual study, it was important because it was a thorough review of the literature on the prevalence and etiology of smoking by adolescent girls and included 35 references that might provide further resources. Caroline included this paper and made a note in the comments column that the authors had reported rates of smoking for teenage girls.

When Caroline finished abstracting all of the articles in the Documents folder, she took the list of additional references she had compiled during the abstracting process and looked each up on MEDLINE. She then repeated the process she had followed earlier of considering whether to include any of these papers in her review. A paper published in 1993 was added. Caroline included this study in the review matrix at the end of the 1993 list and abstracted it as she had done the others.

After completion, Caroline had a review matrix filled in with notes for each article. The matrix was a little messy because there were additional notes on stickies and a few more column topics had been added. She was ready to write the synthesis.

# REFERENCES

1. National Center for Health Statistics. *Health Interview Survey Procedures, 1957–1974.* Hyattsville, MD: U.S. Department of Health, Education, and Welfare, Public Health Service, Health Resources Administration; 1975.

2. Kovar MG, Poe GS. *The National Health Interview Survey Design, 1975–83*. Hyattsville, MD: U.S. Department of Health and Human Services, Public Health Service, National Center for Health Statistics; 1985.

3. Masey JT, Moore TF, Parsons VL, Tadros W. *Design and Estimation for the National Health Interview Survey, 1985–94*. Hyattsville, MD: U.S. Department of Health and Human Services, Public Health Service, Centers for Disease Control, National Center for Health Statistics; 1989.

4. Wang MQ, Fitzhugh EC, Westerfield RC, Eddy JM. Family and peer influences on smoking behavior among American adolescents: an age trend. *J Adoles Health*. 1995;16:200–203.

5. Altman DG, Levine DW, Coeytaux R, Slade J, Jaffe R. Tobacco promotion and susceptibility to tobacco use among adolescents aged 12 through 17 years in a nationally representative sample. *Am J Public Health*. 1996;86:1590–1593.

6. French SA, Perry CL. Smoking among adolescent girls: Prevalence and etiology. *J Am Med Womens Assoc*. 1996;51:25–28.

# 6 Synthesis: How to Use a Review Matrix to Write a Synthesis

The goal of a review of the literature is to summarize your critical analysis about the research literature on a specific topic in the form of a narrative. This chapter describes how to use a review matrix to write such a synthesis and includes the following sections:

- ⊙ What Is a Synthesis?
- ⊙ How to Use a Review Matrix to Write a Synthesis
- ⊙ Caroline's Quest: Writing a Synthesis

# WHAT IS A SYNTHESIS?

A synthesis is a critical analysis and review of the scientific literature on a specific topic. Unlike a summary of different articles, a synthesis is based on the same set of papers and examines the themes of the research as they have developed across the studies and over the years, including similarities and discrepancies in purpose, content, methodology, and findings. A synthesis also examines the literature for what is missing—where the holes are in both the content and the research methodology. The goal of a synthesis is to analyze critically the content of the research, research methodologies, and results and then to pull the disparate parts together into a logical, coherent whole.

## Advantages of a Synthesis

Most people find that they do not formulate interpretations or opinions about the research studies until they have written a systematic review of the literature. A well-written literature review requires that you complete two major tasks: critically analyze the literature and write a synthesis. The operational word here is write. To stop before putting the synthesis into written form will have accomplished only half the task of your literature review.

## What This Chapter Does Not Cover

This chapter is not about how to write. There are excellent books available on that subject, beginning with the classic *If You Want to Write*, by Brenda Ueland.[1] Other excellent guides are *How to Write: Advice and Reflections* by Pulitzer Prize-winning writer Richard Rhodes[2] and *Writing Down the Bones* by award-winning writing instructor Natalie Goldberg.[3] You will also need a good grammar book. A classic is *Elements of Style* by Strunk and White[4]; its witty, contemporary counterpart is *Woe Is I* by Patricia O'Conner.[5] These writing and grammar books are excellent resources, whether you intend to write a synthesis of the literature or any other kind of document.

# HOW TO USE A REVIEW MATRIX TO WRITE A SYNTHESIS

## The Tools You Will Need

After all of the source documents in the Documents folder have been abstracted and the review matrix has been completed, you are ready to begin the synthesis. The review matrix is the primary tool for organizing and writing the synthesis. You will use not only the content in the matrix, but also the tracking information to locate quickly the original articles in the Documents folder. Thus, you will need both the review matrix and the Documents folder close at hand in writing the synthesis.

## Using the Review Matrix

The review matrix has a different use in writing a synthesis than it did for abstracting source documents. Constructing the review matrix required you to develop the rows of the matrix by analyzing one study at a time based on the column topics. In writing a synthesis of the literature, you will focus on the columns of the review matrix as you compare the studies.

Of course you have to know each of the studies, but when you begin to synthesize them, you are looking at them from a different angle. For example, you could think about how the studies varied over time in their use of a particular theory. Alternatively, you might want to identify only those studies that included both male and female subjects. By scanning a particular column of the review matrix, you can readily identify those studies. (It might be easier to sort the studies in your review matrix on the basis of information in one of the columns.) You might also look for the lack of something across the studies. For example, in papers on the epidemiology of epilepsy, did any of the subject populations include people over 65 years of age? If you abstracted information in the review matrix about subjects' age ranges, then you will be able to look for that possibility. In general, as you critically evaluate the different studies, think about the underlying factor that you want to use to show variations or lack thereof over time.

## Reason for the Review

The first step in writing a synthesis is to be clear about why you are doing a literature review. The most common reasons include summarizing previous scholarly work for a paper or report for a class, gathering background material for a presentation or publication; preparing a thesis or dissertation required in a graduate program; writing a research proposal, including a request for grant or contract funds; and writing a scientific article, possibly describing your own research or that of others.

The focus of the literature review will vary, depending on the reason for doing the review. The reason should provide you with guidance in focusing the literature review. In a thesis or dissertation, the previous research section contains most of the review of the literature, whereas the background and significance sections of a standard grant or contract proposal include most of the literature review. In the thesis or dissertation and the research proposal, the review of the literature may focus not only on the major topic, such as previous research on the effects of poor nutrition among lower income children, but also on a methodological review; that is, the types of research methods used by previous researchers in the field to investigate that topic. In a scientific paper, the review of the literature will be most evident in the introduction and discussion sections.

## Define the Purpose of the Review

The next step in writing a synthesis is to define clearly the purpose of the review of the literature. You should have done this already when you began assembling the paper trail; however, that purpose may have changed as you read and reread the source documents. Perhaps the purpose is more refined in scope or has been expanded to encompass more issues. Either way, the first working sentence of your synthesis should be this: "The purpose of this review of the literature is . . ."

## Describe the Search and Review Process

Describe briefly the strategy used to select and review the documents included in your literature review. This description provides basic information about your search and selection process, such as the period of time covered by the review, the sources used, including electronic bibliographic databases and journals, types of articles, and the conditions for inclusions and exclusions. The following example conveys such information:

> The review of the literature covered a ten-year period, from 1990 to 1999. The search included use of three electronic bibliographic databases, MEDLINE, PsychInfo, and International Pharmaceutical Abstracts, with special attention to the leading clinical journals in this area (*Journal of X, Journal of Y,* and *Journal of Z*). Only empirical studies were reviewed; letters to the editor, policy statements, and program descriptions were excluded. A total of 103 papers were examined, of which 23 met the criteria.

Because you are using the Matrix Method, you might also tell the reader what topics were used to abstract the documents. Here is an example:

> Using the Matrix Method,[6] each of the 23 papers was evaluated in ascending chronologic order using a structured abstracting form with 12 topics: journal identification, purpose, definition of independent and dependent variables, covariates, methodological design, sampling design, number of subjects, respondent/nonrespondent analysis, data sources, validity and reliability of data collection, results, and significance.

The description of the search and abstracting process will vary, depending on the purpose of your review. For example, if you are summarizing the literature for a research paper, then the description may need to be more concise. Alternatively, the process used to review the literature for a meta-analysis will need to be more extensive. Regardless of the purpose of your paper, a statement of the search and abstracting process will give the reader a sense of the thoroughness of your literature review.

## List the Principal Topics

Now think about which topics you will use to organize the synthesis. A thorough synthesis of the literature includes a discussion of one or more of the following:

- *Issues*: The major reasons or problems that motivated this body of research, including the theoretical or conceptual models and the hypothesis or research question.

- *Methods*: The research methods used to investigate the problems, including one or more of the column topics, are listed under the broad headings of methodology, data collection instruments and procedures, subjects, and data analysis.
- *Results*: The major findings or results.
- *Missing or inadequate topics*: The topics or issues that are missing, that is, those that have not been investigated at all or those that have been covered inadequately.
- *Critical analysis*: Your critical analysis of each of these sections.

It is important to separate your discussion of the literature, that is, the issues, methods, results, and missing topics, from your critical analysis. Make certain that you specify which is which in your review. Although all five issues are needed, your critical analysis of this body of research is probably the most important. Critical, in this context, is not the same as negative. A critical analysis is one in which you have weighed all of the evidence and made an informed judgment about the adequacy, appropriateness, and thoroughness of the studies reviewed.

You can structure the written synthesis of the literature in several different ways. One approach might be to write up each of the first four sections—issues, methods, missing or inadequate, and results—and at the end of each of those sections give a critical analysis.

Another approach would be to summarize the first four topics together and conclude with a section containing the critical analysis. Often the decision about how to structure a review of the literature will be made after you have written the first draft, not at the beginning of the process. In fact, you might choose the structure only after revising the review several times.

Alternatively, the reason for doing the review may dictate the structure and format of your synthesis. For example, a synthesis written for a doctoral dissertation will be very different from one prepared for a research study manuscript being submitted to a peer-reviewed journal.

## Read the Columns

With the purpose, topics, and structure of your written synthesis in mind, how do you use the review matrix to synthesize the information? Read each of the columns of the matrix from top to bottom and determine what happened within each topic heading across the studies and over time. For example, if you are summarizing the themes of the research studies, look down the purpose column in the review matrix. Are there specific issues that appear, disappear, and then reappear over the years?

If it is necessary to gather more details, go back and reread some of the papers, which you already will have arranged in convenient, chronologic order in the Documents folder in the Lit Review master folder. Having abstracted all of the articles, you should have developed a sense of how thoroughly the various authors reviewed other studies by their inclusion of citations to published papers. Did these authors refer to other studies? Alternatively, did other authors seem to strike out on their own, without referring to the work of previous research that could have been used to better develop their own ideas? Taken as a body of research, does this collection of articles suggest that many different themes were addressed over the period you reviewed, or does this set of articles focus on one central theme, with the studies building on one another?

Do the papers seem to concentrate on increasingly specific details about the same issue, with only a few that explore new areas of inquiry? Is this an appropriate, creative, or necessary diversion from the mainstream of research on the subject? If you are developing ideas for your own research, perhaps in the form of a dissertation or research proposal, what holes are there that you might focus on in this body of research?

The same kind of thinking could be applied to the methodologies used to examine the research questions. Are the studies merely descriptive, or do subsequent studies describe innovative approaches for solving the problem? For example, in the research literature on falls among older women, initial papers described high prevalence rates that often resulted in the women's confinement to a nursing home or in their death. Later papers reported a statistical association between falls and use of antianxiety drugs, with the conclusion that these medications were overused in the older population. In subsequent papers, only a subclass of antianxiety drugs was found to be the problem. Next was a series of studies that described the effects of different methods for intervening with practicing physicians to convince them to change their prescription of these drugs, especially for older people. Taken as a whole, this body of research moved from the initial description of the problem, through association with risk factors, to intervention. The corresponding methodological designs used in these studies followed a similar progression from descriptive to quasiexperimental to experimental designs.

After completing the synthesis, you will need to store a final copy of your review of the literature in the synthesis section of the Lit Review master folder for later reference.

# Caroline's Quest: Writing a Synthesis

Caroline met with Professor Dickerson to go over her review matrix and discuss the next steps.

"Keep in mind why you are writing this synthesis," Professor Dickerson cautioned her. "The way you write the review, its length, and issues you cover may vary depending on whether the synthesis is being written for a term paper, a thesis, or a grant proposal. In this case, you know it is the introductory section for your thesis, but in the future, your purpose will vary."

Caroline understood his point but had a question about her immediate task. "I'd like to talk about how to organize the synthesis itself. You know, what do I discuss first, then next, and so forth?"

Professor Dickerson nodded and said, "I know what you mean. The first thing to remember is that you should not merely summarize each paper. Instead, think about the issues you want to describe. Certainly you will be describing information from each study, but your focus should be on a critical analysis of the major aspects of research that these studies cover. You might begin your synthesis by describing the purpose of your review and limitations that you chose, such as a focus on adolescent girls between the ages of 13 and 18 years old. You could also include a few sentences on the search itself, the years you restricted it to, the databases you searched, and the number of articles you included in the review. All of this is preliminary to your actual synthesis, however, and should probably not take more than half a page. Concentrate the remainder of your synthesis on the critical analysis of the studies.

"For example," he continued, "think about the different kinds of research questions that the authors asked in their studies. Were there any major themes? If so, describe them briefly. Summarize the major findings, and then discuss how the studies differed in what they found. In general, think about using the following strategy: summarize the issue, describe variations across the studies, discuss strengths and weaknesses of the studies, and give your interpretation about what this means."

Caroline looked at the materials she had brought with her. "So how do I use the review matrix in writing the synthesis?" she asked. "Or is preparing the review matrix just a way of making me read each article in a disciplined fashion?"

"Good question," Professor Dickerson responded. "You're right. Filling in the review matrix does make you read each study carefully and make notes on the same set of topics, but the review matrix is also very useful in two other ways in the actual writing of the synthesis. The matrix helps you think about which topics to cover in the synthesis. The organization of the synthesis you write will not be identical to the column topics listed across the top of your review matrix, but those column topics may help you think about which issues to include."

Professor Dickerson pointed to Caroline's review matrix on her laptop. "The most practical way to use the review matrix is to read down each column and think about how the studies vary or how they are alike. For example, look at the variations in number of subjects across the studies."

Caroline reexamined the review matrix she had prepared and began to see the variations Professor Dickerson was talking about. "I hadn't realized how much the studies differed," she commented. "At first they all looked pretty much alike. Actually, when I began doing this review of the literature, I had the sense that there was nothing left to study. It seemed like all of the research questions had been asked and answered."

Professor Dickerson smiled and replied, "Yes, that's the sense most people have when they first begin to read the scientific literature on a specific topic. By constructing a review matrix, however, you begin to see where the holes are. The review matrix helps you realize which areas appear to be missing and which topics have been covered pretty thoroughly."

"But it is important," he cautioned, "if you see what you think is an area or aspect that is missing, then try to find other studies in which the missing topic has been studied. In other words, is it missing because no one has studied that aspect of the field, or is it because you didn't do a thorough enough job of finding all the studies?"

"Okay, I understand," Caroline looked at her professor and continued in a firm voice, "But this afternoon, I have to write the first draft of the synthesis for my thesis. What do I begin with? Then what do I write next? How do I organize this synthesis?"

Professor Dickerson took out a blank sheet of paper and made some notes as he talked. "Keep in mind that the organization will vary depending on your purpose. But as we discussed before, one structure you could use might be the following: describe the purpose of your literature review; summarize briefly the characteristics of the search process; describe the structure you are going to follow in writing this synthesis—in other words, the topics you are going to summarize—discuss the similarities and differences across the studies under each topic; and finally, describe your interpretation of what this means. In your interpretation, state your opinion, based on your logical and critical analysis of the literature. Include your thoughts about what is known based on this research, what hasn't been adequately covered, and what is missing. If you have some suggestions about how you would address these inadequacies, then describe them. In writing the section on your interpretation, be sure to make it clear that these are your opinions and not those of the authors of the papers."

Caroline gathered together her papers and prepared to leave. "I feel that I really know this literature," she said. "Well, I have a good sense of what this set of articles covers, anyway," she amended. "For me, the review matrix was most helpful in making me concentrate on the same set of topics in reading each paper."

Professor Dickerson nodded and replied, "You'll also find that the review matrix is very helpful in the writing process too. I'll be interested in seeing how your first draft of the synthesis turns out."

# REFERENCES

1. Ueland B. *If You Want to Write*. 10th ed. St. Paul, MN: Graywolf; 1997.
2. Rhodes R. *How to Write: Advice and Reflections*. New York, NY: William Morrow and Company; 1996.
3. Goldberg N. *Writing Down the Bones: Freeing the Writer Within*. Boston, MA: Shambhala; 1986.
4. Strunk W, White EB. *Elements of Style*. New York, NY: Macmillan; 1979.
5. O'Conner PT. *Woe Is I: The Grammarphobe's Guide to Better English in Plain English*. East Rutherford, NJ: Putnam; 1996.
6. Garrard J. *Health Sciences Literature Review Made Easy: The Matrix Method*. 3rd ed. Sudbury, MA: Jones and Bartlett; 2010.

Part

# III Applications Using the Matrix Method

# 7 A Library of Lit Review Master Folders

Creating a lit review master folder is a first step in the Matrix Method, but if you have conducted literature reviews for two or more different subjects, then how do you manage multiple master folders? The purpose of this chapter is to describe what a library of lit review master folders is and why it is worth developing and maintaining. The concept, which is simple, gives you the efficiency to buy yourself time in the future. The Matrix Method tells you how to conduct a review of the literature; this chapter tells you what to do afterwards. The sections of this chapter are as follows:

- ⊙ What Is a Library of Lit Review Master Folders?
- ⊙ How to Create a Library of Lit Review Master Folders
- ⊙ How to Use a Library of Lit Review Master Folders
- ⊙ Making the Most of the Matrix Method
- ⊙ Caroline's Quest: Building Her Own Library of Master Folders

# WHAT IS A LIBRARY OF LIT REVIEW MASTER FOLDERS?

Suppose that over the past few years you have completed not one, but five lit reviews for different subjects. For each of these literature reviews, you have created a complete lit review master folder, with the four sub-folders described earlier in this book. You now have a library of lit review master folders consisting of a collection of computer folders on your desktop. Even one lit review master folder makes a library. Just storing lit review master folders, however, is not sufficient. This is a resource that is useful only if two additional conditions are met: the lit review master folders are updated periodically, and you create and use some kind of indexing system so that you know what is available. The purpose of this chapter is to describe how to use a collection of lit review master folders. The next chapter describes how to index the information they contain.

## Advantages of a Library of Lit Review Master Folders

If you organize your master folders as a library, then you buy yourself time which can be a scarce resource. With a master folders library, you also gain the practical advantage of not having to duplicate previous efforts to find and download a copy of an article or source document. In the initial review of the literature, you make a one-time investment in time and effort. By creating and maintaining a library of lit review master folders, you will benefit from the interest on that investment in the future.

# HOW TO CREATE A LIBRARY OF LIT REVIEW MASTER FOLDERS

A literature review usually is done in a flurry of activity, with an intense effort focused on getting the synthesis written and the product produced, whether it is a paper, a grant proposal, or a final report. Afterwards, the by-products of this effort are set aside—the downloaded articles in the Documents folder, the notes in the Paper Trail folder, the review matrix in its folder, and final written product in the Synthesis folder. They are accumulated in the Lit Review master folder until they are needed again. Usually the impetus for returning to a lit review master folder is the need for a particular source document that you know was part of the initial review.

## Adopt a Labeling Convention

The secret to being efficient in the future is knowing where your lit review master folders are and keeping them up to date. Your first task is to assign a label to each of your lit review master folders. For example, create a label based on the subject of your lit review: Epilepsy Lit Review master folder, or Maternal and Child Health Lit Review master folder. Next, store them all together in a folder of master folders. You might call this folder your Master Folders Library.

Take this labeling of folders one step further by using the same label for the four subfolders that make up the master folder. For example, in the Epilepsy master folder, create an Epilepsy Paper Trail folder, an Epilepsy Documents folder, an Epilepsy Matrix folder, and an Epilepsy Synthesis folder. By using the same label, you can search your documents just on the label alone to find them all.

Detailed instructions for how to set up a structure of computer folders for the Matrix Method are given in Appendix B, together with answers to frequently asked questions about this strategy.

## Keep the Master Folders Up to Date

Keeping your lit review master folders up to date is another practice that takes time and self-discipline. As you come across new studies, download a copy of the article to the Documents folder in the appropriate lit review master folder. An alternative is to let new documents accumulate in a safe place and at some later point, file them in the documents folders in the appropriate lit review master folders.

Expanding a documents folder is not the only reason for updating a lit review master folder. Additions to the paper trail might include new, topical websites or lecture notes from subsequent courses. Consider setting aside one part of the paper trail to store notes from scientific meetings you attended after the synthesis was written. You do not have to know exactly how you will use these added materials in the future, but you do need a dependable storage system in order to find them when you need them. A library of updated lit review master folders provides such a system.

## HOW TO USE A LIBRARY OF LIT REVIEW MASTER FOLDERS

An updated library of lit review master folders can be very useful as you progress through your student or professional career as a catalog over time. Simply finding things is a fundamental problem; trying to find things you know you have but cannot lay your hands on is a frustrating, fundamental problem. A library of lit review master folders provides a permanent storage system that you can use from course to course and year to year.

A second use is that of integrating information across topics or content areas. Whether you are a graduate student, researcher, policy analyst, or writer, you will inevitably find yourself doing more than one review of the literature. Even when your literature review is on a single topic, you may find it necessary to delve into several different subjects, possibly with a review and synthesis of each. For example, if you are conducting research on the effects of penicillin as a treatment for ear infections in children, you might need to review the literature on the clinical effectiveness of penicillin and later conduct a separate review on ear infections and still later do a third review of papers on research methodologies used to study patient outcomes of clinical treatment. For each of these topics you could create a separate lit review master folder, especially if the review has a complex paper trail or a large number of source documents in the Documents folder. Your review of studies on the treatment of ear infections then might result in three lit review master folders—one labeled Penicillin Treatment; a second, Ear Infections; and a third, Research Methods.

After completion of the synthesis on penicillin treatment, you might use the Lit Review master folder on research methods as your central file for methodological papers and notes. Thus, a lit review master folder created for one review could be useful in a multitude of other reviews.

A library of lit review master folders that has been kept up to date can be a valuable resource for a group of people, such as a research team or collaborators on a project. A library can serve as a central archive, making it easier for team members to store and find commonly used materials. This also has the advantage of increasing the opportunity for shared knowledge. Let the rules for keeping the library up to date be simple; anyone can add an article or source document to the appropriate lit review master folder in the library, but the same person also has to take the responsibility of notifying other team members about the new addition by posting the addition in an indexing system on a server or updating the printed list in the Documents folder. A central archive buys time and effort for the team and reduces the necessity of downloading multiple copies and storing in each individual's lit review master folder.

# MAKING THE MOST OF THE MATRIX METHOD

By now, you probably understand the basic concepts about how to use the Matrix Method. But bear in mind that a successfully completed review of the literature may not always follow exactly the instructions in the previous chapters. Exhibit 7-1 describes some of the concepts and the variations that may be useful to the experienced user of the Matrix Method. These are given in the form of answers to questions about how to get the most out of the Matrix Method.

| Exhibit | |
|---|---|
| **7-1** | How to Get the Most out of the Matrix Method |

WHY DO I HAVE TO READ AN ARTICLE
MULTIPLE TIMES IN THE MATRIX METHOD?

You read for different purposes. You need to read an article or source document at least three times. Here is a summary of each reading (and the chapters that describe the purpose for each).

- **First Reading: Select Document.** The first time you read a source document (an article or paper in a journal) is to decide whether it is relevant to your

*(continues)*

| Exhibit | |
|---|---|
| **7-1** | **Continued** |

topic. This initial reading may be just of the abstract or a skimming of the article. For example, read the title and abstract in the bibliographic database (e.g., PubMed) to determine relevancy to your topic. You may select or discard potential articles at this stage, but try to be as broad in your choices as possible. This first reading does not have to be in chronologic order by publication date. The end product is a set of downloaded articles or pdf files in your documents folder. (Chapter 4).

- **Second Reading: Column Topics**. This reading is for purposes of deciding what column topics to include in the review matrix. By this point you have selected a large number of articles (or other source documents). Organize them in chronologic order, from oldest to most recent, and begin this reading with the oldest. Reread the abstract and the entire article, making a list of potential column topics as you go. The end product at this stage is an empty review matrix with column topics listed across the top (and room for more to be added). (Chapter 5).

- **Third Reading: Critical Review**. At this stage, you read each article thoroughly and abstract it based on the column topics. This is your first critical review of the article, and you approach it with a calculator and electronic sticky notes or other ways of making notes in the document itself. Read the article section by section, and make notes in the cells of the review matrix (as well as copious notes on the article itself as you record your thoughts). (Exhibit 5-1 in Chapter 5). The end product should be a filled-in review matrix with the column topics across the top and all the articles listed in chronologic order (oldest to most recent) down the side.

- **Later Readings: Compare**. A fourth, fifth, and sixth reading may be necessary as you develop your understanding of the literature you are reviewing. These later readings may be necessary as you compare an article with others. Examples of these comparisons could be about the purpose of the study, the number of subjects who completed the treatment, or the authors' interpretation of significance of the findings. (Note the sections, "To Own the Literature" in Chapter 1 and "Seeing What Is Missing" in Chapter 5). While drawing these comparisons, you're creating the first draft of your synthesis.

## How Many Articles Are Enough?

This is a common question, and my answer is always the same: "It depends." You need to abstract enough articles that you feel you own the literature (Chapter 1). If only a few papers have been published about your topic, then this may be a signal that you need to broaden your topic. If there are too many, e.g., 100 or more, then narrow your focus, perhaps by selecting only studies with more stringent methodological designs (such as only those with an experimental design or those with more than 25 subjects in a group). If you are examining studies of a specific drug treatment and there are too few published, then consider whether this drug is one of a broader class of drugs. Including more publications about the treatment effects of that broader class may help put this drug into perspective.

## How Far Back Do I Go in the Literature and When Do I Use an Old, Old Article?

While you are reviewing abstracts in the selection process (the first reading), pay close attention to which publications those articles are referencing. As you become more familiar with research papers about your topic, it is likely that you will notice that the research of some of the same authors are being referenced repeatedly by others. Conduct an author search in your bibliographic database (e.g., PubMed), identify which of that author's papers are related to your topic, and look at the dates of those publications. If the dates are older than the ones you have included thus far, then include them, and let the oldest of these be designated as your oldest publication.

Sometimes it is possible to recognize frequently referenced authors before the abstracting process begins, and the search for papers about those can be started before you develop your review matrix. That is the preferred strategy and allows you to begin the abstracting process from a logical beginning. If not, be alert for frequently referenced authors, and include them at whatever stage of the abstracting process you discover them.

A related problem is when you find a paper in the peer-reviewed literature that is quite old compared to the papers you have already selected. If that really old paper is closely related to your topic, then consider the possibility that there are other papers you haven't found yet in between the oldest date and the date your other papers begin. Go back and look for them; perhaps this is the point to try using the Science Citation Index based on a search under each author's name. (See a description of Science Citation Index in the Chapter 3 section, "How to Find Source Materials:

*(continues)*

| Exhibit | |
|---|---|
| **7-1** | **Continued** |

Creating and Using a Paper Trail.") If you don't find any papers in between the two dates, then perhaps there are none, but include that oldest paper anyway.

### WHAT DO I DO ABOUT QUALITATIVE STUDIES?

A qualitative study can be thought of as one that does not include statistical analysis, mainly because the results do not lend themselves to quantitative procedures. Qualitative results can have a powerful impact on the interpretation of data that cannot be gathered any other way. For example, if a researcher is studying the impact of a new federal policy on quality of life of nursing home elderly, then one kind of study would be to ask nursing home residents about the positive and negative aspects of living there. Do this before and after the policy has been implemented. A comparison of responses from those prepost periods may be very useful. Another example would be a content analysis of interview data in qualitative research about treatment effects of a new medical device. A content analysis can be a rigorous nonquantitative method for systematically examining variations in interview data. See an example of the use of content analysis in a study my colleagues and I did of organizational change in the management of hepatitis C.[1]

If some of the articles describe qualitative research and others quantitative research, should they be included in the same review matrix? How do we draw conclusions from such a mixture of quantitative and qualitative research? There is no definite rule about this. My tendency would be to separate the quantitative and qualitative studies, use the same column headings if possible, and then add new ones for the qualitative studies. Examples of column topics that would be the same for both might be number of subjects, data collection instrument, validity and reliability studies of data collection instrument, sampling method, and methodological design. New columns to be added for the qualitative studies might include details about how data were collected, e.g., focus group, telephone interview, and how data were analyzed.

In writing the synthesis, examine the results of the two review matrices (quantitative and qualitative research) separately. You may find that one complements or enriches the other. Alternatively, combine all the studies in a single, chronologically arranged review matrix, regardless of quantitative or qualitative characteristics, and summarize these results.

In general, as research methods have become more sophisticated over time, many scientists use both kinds of research, and it is very difficult to characterize a study as solely quantitative or qualitative.

## How Do I Review and Abstract Longitudinal Studies?

Longitudinal studies are those that collect data from subjects at multiple points over a long period of time, where researchers can define *long* in different ways, such as multiple weeks, months, or years.

Publications about longitudinal studies can vary in several ways; the primary author may differ, the research site may not be the same, the research question may vary around a principal topic, the purpose of the paper may change (for example, some may describe new methodological developments, whereas others may concentrate on clinical outcomes), and the year of publication of the paper varies over time. If all of these studies clearly show that there was a core research team with a primary research goal, then here is a suggestion for abstracting these studies. Set aside a section of the review matrix and abstract them in their chronologic order (from oldest to most recent) using the same column topics as in the rest of your review matrix. This arrangement will give you the opportunity to consider that subset of research as a whole, rather than as a collection of discrete studies that happened to have some commonalities. If there are multiple longitudinal studies, perhaps from researchers based in different countries, then you will be in a better position to describe these research endeavors as a group and perhaps understand what the literature is saying about your topic.

## How Can Matrices Be Combined and Why Should They Be?

The Matrix Method has been described as the activity by one person who is reviewing the literature on a specific topic. This method can be extended to use by two or more people with two or more topics. Here is an example. Suppose a clinical outcomes research group in a large, managed care organization needed to review the literature about a medical device that became available on the market ten years ago. The goal of this team was to understand what the research has to say about the clinical effectiveness of the medical device for use by patients. The organization's clinical board was interested in possibly recommending the device to clinicians in its network. The research team consisted of a physician, nurse practitioner, biostatistician, epidemiologist, and consumer advocate. All were accomplished in the use of the Matrix Method, RefWorks, which was their organization's reference management software, and a variety of electronic bibliographic databases such as MEDLINE and CINAHL. Should one of these team members review the literature and summarize the results for the others? What would be the benefit if they all reviewed the literature? If all participated in the review, how would they divide up the work?

*(continues)*

| Exhibit | |
|---|---|
| **7-1** | **Continued** |

The team decided that each of them would review the literature because they all needed to be at the same level of understanding of research about the device. They began by discussing the purpose of the review, then each would apply the Matrix Method separately and compare their progress at these stages: (1) selection of articles, (2) creation of the column topics, (3) completion of the review matrix, and (4) draft of the synthesis. They agreed at the beginning that each reviewer would have a different focus: the physician would concentrate on clinical outcomes and medical factors related to its use, the nurse practitioner would focus on patient factors that contributed to success or failure of the device; the biostatistician would be responsible for evaluating the methods and statistical procedures and explaining the statistical outcomes to the group; the epidemiologist would be concerned about population findings about use in different settings (home, community, nursing home), in different geographic areas, and under other conditions in which the device was used; and the consumer advocate would focus on patient reactions and evaluations about ease of use in everyday life. Team members set about the task separately in identifying articles and creating column topics.

The reason the team members compared their results at four points was to standardize the review. The final selection of articles to be reviewed were those collected by all team members. They realized that some articles might not be relevant to their focus, but all team members would have to summarize each article by its purpose, methods, and relevance to the general purpose. This meant that when one team member described a study, they all were familiar with the content. The discussion of the column topics also reflected all of their input. They used a decision rule of agreeing on general topics such as purpose, methods, description of data collection instruments, methodological design, and statistical procedures.

Then each had a section specific to his or her own focus. Everybody had a final column in which they could record their impression of the study. Each completed the review matrix separately. They went over the results of these review matrices in a discussion section and agreed on the outline and content of the synthesis. Each drafted the synthesis for his/her own focus. The result was a document that reflected all of their investment in time and effort, their expertise, and their focus, and they agreed on the recommendations to the board.

In another example, a class of students took a similar approach when they divided up into teams of five and used the Matrix Method to review the same topic, but worked separately until they came together to prepare the synthesis based on their separately prepared review matrices.

A third example is given in Chapter 9 in the section, "How to Use Matrix Applications in Practice Guidelines."

### WHAT IS PLAGIARISM?

Plagiarism is claiming the work of others as your own. Books, articles, and websites have discussed this problem at length. The focus here is to describe how to avoid it in the context of the Matrix Method. Always put quotation marks around any material you copy directly from a source document and record the citation at the end of the quote. When you are preparing the synthesis of the review of the literature, describe the quoted material in your own words. It is still necessary to show where the ideas (written in your own words) came from.

# Caroline's Quest:
# Building Her Own Library of Master Folders

In addition to working on her master's thesis, Caroline also had several term papers to write in some of her other courses. In her developmental psychology course, Caroline reviewed the literature on differences in self-esteem between male and female adolescents. Some of the research articles she included in that review were the same papers she had included in her thesis.

Caroline wanted to create a reprint file that she could maintain during and after her graduate school program. Professor Dickerson suggested that she set up a reprint filing system around a library of lit review master folders with a documents folder in each. Because she planned to have multiple lit review master folders, she assigned the same label to each of the four folders within each master folder. For example, the Self-Esteem Lit Review master folder included the Self-Esteem Paper Trail folder, the Self-Esteem Documents folder, the Self-Esteem Review Matrix folder, and the Self-Esteem Synthesis folder. For her thesis lit review she created the

Adolescent Smoking Lit Review master folder, which included the following four folders: Adolescent Smoking Paper Trail folder, Adolescent Smoking Documents folder, Adolescent Smoking Review Matrix folder, and Adolescent Smoking Synthesis folder.

Caroline used the self-esteem and smoking article both in the paper she wrote for the course on adolescent development and in her thesis. The paper was filed only once, however, in the Self-Esteem Documents folder because it was created before she began reviewing the literature for her thesis. By using the Matrix Indexing System, described in the next chapter, Caroline was able to keep track of whether she had a copy of an article and where each was filed.

Over the two years of her graduate program, Caroline accumulated six lit review master folders, including one on research methods and another on public health interventions. Depending on which subject each lit review master folder covered, she included notes from national meetings and government reports. Some of these additions were included after the literature review was completed. These master folders were stored in her master folders library, a library that grew over the years as she added new articles and documents from her work. An important part of maintaining that library was keeping an up-to-date record of the materials she had and where they were stored. Thus, an integral part of creating and using a master folders library is its integration with the Matrix Indexing System, described in the next chapter.

# REFERENCE

1. Garrard J, Choudary V, Groom H, et al. Organizational change in management of hepatitis C: Evaluation of a CME program. *J Contin Educ Health Prof.* 2006;26(2):145–160.

# 8 The Matrix Indexing System

The Matrix Indexing System described in this chapter consists of merging information from three different sources: electronic bibliographic databases, reference management software, and the documents folders within one or more lit review master folders. The topics covered in this chapter are as follows:

- ⊙ What Is the Matrix Indexing System?
- ⊙ How to Set up a Matrix Indexing System
- ⊙ How to Expand the Documents Folder
- ⊙ How to Update a Literature Review Efficiently
- ⊙ Caroline's Quest: Using the Matrix Indexing System

# WHAT IS THE MATRIX INDEXING SYSTEM?

How do you create a system for organizing materials across multiple reviews of the literature, over time as you add new source documents, and share these with colleagues or associates? The Matrix Indexing System was developed for just these purposes. It is a plan for organizing your references and documents and managing this information on an ongoing basis. This indexing system can be useful throughout a professional career whether you begin using it as a student or later in your career.

The Matrix Indexing System consists of these activities:

- Merging information from three sources: (1) an electronic bibliographic database such as MEDLINE, (2) reference management software such as RefWorks, EndNote, or ProCite, and (3) the Documents folder within your Lit Review master folder
- Expanding the Documents folder in your Lit Review master folder
- Updating a review of the literature

## Advantages of a Matrix Indexing System

If you set up your initial review of the literature using the Matrix Method, then you already have a start on the Matrix Indexing System. However, the indexing system differs from the Matrix Method. The Matrix Method is a strategy for acquiring, analyzing, and writing a synthesis of a review of the scientific literature. In contrast, the Matrix Indexing System provides a way of coping with all the information and documents that you use or create as a result of a review of the literature. In other words, the Matrix Indexing System gives you a way to create a manageable system in the afterlife of each review of the literature. This chapter explains how to create and use the Matrix Indexing System.

# HOW TO SET UP A MATRIX INDEXING SYSTEM

You need four tools in order to create a Matrix Indexing System: electronic bibliographic databases, reference management software, source documents downloaded in the Documents folder, and location labels.

## Electronic Bibliographic Databases

From your own computer, you must be able to access one or more of the electronic bibliographic databases, such as MEDLINE or CINAHL, or any of those listed in Exhibit 3-2. A dozen or more electronic bibliographic databases are available to health sciences professionals, and more are being created at a rapid rate. MEDLINE is the oldest and largest of these databases in the health sciences. Check with the reference librarian at a biomedical library about new databases that have come online in recent months. An example of a source of electronic bibliographic databases can be seen at the University of Minnesota libraries site, http://www.lib.umn.edu/site/free.phtml, which lists electronic indexes for a very large number of subjects. In this context, the term *index* is used interchangeably with *database*. The indexes at this universal resource locator (URL) are available free to the public.

An effort is also under way by the National Science Foundation to encourage the development and use of electronic libraries. Their availability over the coming years might offer additional resources to professionals in the health sciences. Check out further information on the National Library of Medicine at http://gateway.nlm.nih.gov/gw/Cmd.

In describing the role of an electronic bibliographic database in the Matrix Indexing System, MEDLINE is used as the example, although this indexing system applies to any of the databases described in Chapter 3 and probably to those that have not yet become available.

## Reference Management Software

For your own computer, you need to purchase and install reference management software, such as EndNote or ProCite. If your institution has a subscription to the Web-based product RefWorks, then you can set up your own free database of references—contact your institution's librarian to find out more about this option. Currently, all of these packages (EndNote, ProCite, and RefWorks) have the capability to download information from an electronic bibliographic database to files on users' computers. Further information about EndNote can be found at http://www.endnote.com; information on ProCite is found at http://www.procite.com, and details about RefWorks can be found at http://www.refworks.com. You only need one of these reference management software packages. In choosing that one, you need to ask yourself whether or not you can use it over a long period of time. For example, if you choose RefWorks because your university library has a site license and offers it free to students over the Internet, then find out from the librarian what the rules are for continuting to use RefWorks after you graduate or leave the university. You may have to pay a monthly fee for continued use, but this may be worth the cost.

Software packages designed to format references in research papers and reports have been available for approximately 15 years, and those on the market can be used with a variety of computer platforms, such as Macintosh, PC, and Unix-based systems. They are also known as bibliographic management or citation management software.

## Organizing and Printing References

You can organize references to scientific papers, books, and other source documents cited in scientific or other academic publications and arrange them in the references section of a scientific paper according to your choice of bibliographic style—this is the reference management part of these software packages. The software packages offer numerous bibliographic styles to choose from, including American Psychological Association, the Vancouver style used by many medical journals, Modern Language Association of America, Nature, Proceedings of the National Academy of Science, and the Turabian Reference List style based on the book A Manual for Writers of Term Papers, Theses, and Dissertations.[1]

In preparing a manuscript to be submitted to a journal or for a report or thesis, there is an enormous savings in time and effort in being able to switch from one bibliographic style, such as the style for JAMA in the medical field to another style such as that for the American Psychologist in formatting the references section. This capability alone is reason enough to put a reference management software package on your computer. Over time, however, these packages have developed additional features that are now put to use in the Matrix Indexing System.

## Downloading References and Abstracts

Reference management software packages provide a link between the electronic bibliographic databases, located elsewhere, such as in a biomedical library or on the Internet, to a reference library on your own computer. Reference management software such as EndNote or

RefWorks uses the term *reference library*. In the Matrix Method, this reference library is the same as the Documents folder. With the reference management software, you can download references, including abstracts of journal articles, directly from the electronic databases such as MEDLINE to your computer, which means you do not have to retype the information or paste it on your computer—the software does it for you. If you have difficulty downloading references and abstracts from your library, check with a reference librarian about the possibility of special instructions. Often university-based libraries conduct tutorials about how to use reference management software packages; check to see whether such classes are available at your library.

## *Your Reference Library = Documents Folder*

You can create and maintain one or more user-specified reference libraries (documents folders) on your computer—the software sets these libraries up for you. Read the manual included with the software package.

You can sort references in your Documents folder by author, year of publication, journal, topic, or any other category you specify. Most reference management programs also have a search capability that enables you to find articles within the references you have stored using whatever terms you choose. For example, you can find all of the articles in your own ProCite library that mention the words *randomized clinical trial*.

There is also flexibility about where you will search in your Documents folder. For example, you can direct the search to include the document title, the abstract, and notes you have written about the article. This is a real advantage because the likelihood of finding a source document will be increased if you include a search of the abstract. This search feature is a good reason for always downloading an abstract from the electronic bibliographic database rather than restricting yourself to just the author's name, article title, and journal issue. The manual for the software package explains how to do this.

In addition to searching each reference in the information downloaded from the electronic bibliographic database into your own Documents folder, you can also create your own key words or labels, store these labels in a particular part of the reference file, and then search on those labels. Some of the programs have set aside sections just for this purpose. For example, three such sections provided in EndNote are labels, key words, and notes. You have to decide which section to use consistently as a place for storing your location label for each article.

These two features, storing a key word in a specific location and the search capability, are especially useful in using a standard list of location labels to keep track of where your source documents can be found.

### Reprints in the Documents Folder

You need a documents folder within a lit review master folder from one or more reviews of the literature. Because organization is critical to being able to find things when you need them, think of your Lit Review master folder as residing on a shelf in your office.

### Location Labels for Lit Review Master Folders

Location labels describe where you keep your reprints or other source documents. These location labels provide a link between the references in your reference management software and the reprints in the documents folders in one or more lit review master folders. In creating a standard list of location labels, the most efficient strategy is to make this list before you do a review of the literature or accumulate reprints in the Documents folder in the Lit Review master folder. This means that you will need to use the reference management software package from the beginning. For example, at the initial stage of the review of the literature, as you search the electronic databases for relevant papers in research journals, you can download the references and their corresponding abstracts of interesting papers into your Documents folder. By the time you have completed the review of the literature, you will probably have a large set of references in your Documents folder, only some of which have corresponding reprints, which are also located in the Documents folder in your Lit Review master folder.

Create a list of location labels by tagging each reference in your Documents folder that has a reprint or copy in the Documents folder within your Lit Review master folder. Use a standard label, such as Reprint—Name of lit review master folder. For example, suppose that you have three lit review master folders: one on antidepressants, another on depression, and a third on research methods. Use a location label for each of the downloaded copies of journal articles. The location label for the first lit review master folder would be "Reprint—Antidepressants," those in the second would be labeled "Reprint—Depression," and those in the third, "Reprint—Research Methods." By always putting these labels in a specific location in the reference file, such as the notes section or the label section, or whatever category is available in the computer package you use, you can search these categories for specific key words to find where you stored any reprint you have in your lit review master folders. An example of adding this tag to the label section of a reference in EndNote is shown in Exhibit 8-1.

| Exhibit | |
| --- | --- |
| 8-1 | **Standard Label in an EndNote File about a Reprint in the Documents Folder of a Lit Review Master Folder on Depression** |

**Author**
Smith, Harriet
**Year**
1997
**Title**
Differences between psychotherapy and tricyclic antidepressants in the treatment of depression
**Journal**
*Journal of Treatment*
**Volume**
67
**Issue**
15
**Pages**
1203–1208
**Label**
Reprint—Depression
**Key words**
depression, antidepressants, psychotherapy
**Abstract**
This was a randomized, clinical trial of psychotherapy and tricyclic antidepressants in which 100 female outpatients in a managed care organization were evaluated weekly on a prepost basis. The study period was 1 year, and assessment with the . . .
**Notes**
Excellent methodological design with sufficient numbers of subjects ranging in age from 21 to 64 years. Results show that . . .

*Source*: Courtesy of Thomson Scientific, Inc.

## Location Labels for Materials Not Stored in the Documents Folder

You may not have a downloaded copy of all of the documents that you abstracted in your review matrix. Some documents may be in the form of books or chapters or reports available in your own library. Other source documents may be located elsewhere, such as those in a departmental library or a regional library. These materials may even be too long to be photocopied, despite their usefulness in your review of the literature. For example, a chapter in a standard statistics book might be the key reference that describes an important analytic technique.

Location labels can help you to remember what these references are and where they are located. Keep track of these references by creating a set of labels analogous to the Reprint—lit review master folder label. For example, instead of using the name of a lit review master folder in the label, you might choose another standard set of words, such as *reprint—own library* or *reprint—biomedical library*. Thus, a label such as "Reprint—Own Library" for the statistics book located on the shelf in your office might be the standard label that you use to find the chapter with the analytic technique. The word *reprint* is a useful common tag because it enables you to sort all references on that word alone and thus find the documents quickly and efficiently.

## How the Elements Are Linked

Location labels, together with reference management software, are the keys to managing an overwhelming amount of detail about pdf files, print, or other materials accumulated in a literature review. You might store such a list in a specific section in the Paper Trail folder within your Lit Review master folder. If nothing else, tape a copy of your list of location labels to the back of your office door. The point is to create and use location labels as part of the Matrix Indexing System in order to manage the materials that you accumulate, use intensively, and then leave and forget about but need to access quickly at a later date.

An illustration of how the different elements of a Matrix Indexing System are linked by the reference management software and the location labels is summarized in Figure 8-1. Specifically, references and abstracts of journal articles and other materials are downloaded from an

## Figure 8-1

How Elements in the Matrix Indexing System Are Linked Together

| **Elements of the Matrix Indexing System** | Electronic Bibliographic Database | Your Reference Library on Your Computer | Documents Section of a Lit Review Book |
|---|---|---|---|

| **Linkages Between Elements** | Reference Management Software | Location Labels Stored in the Reference Library on Your Computer |
|---|---|---|

electronic bibliographic database, such as MEDLINE, into your Documents folder on your computer using reference management software such as RefWorks. Using the same reference management software, you create a standard list of location labels and tag each reference in your Documents folder with its location. The advantage of storing all of your reprints chronologically in a documents folder within a lit review master folder and then keeping track of the references in your reference library using location labels is that you will be able to find these materials when you need them. Thus, you create an organized storage and filing system for your reprints, rather than a random collection of articles that you cannot access because you cannot remember what is there or how to locate the materials you need.

## HOW TO EXPAND THE DOCUMENTS FOLDER

As the number of reprints you download increases, you will inevitably be faced with the problem of running information overload. One way of managing this problem is to create a new master folder with another title. For example, suppose your initial literature review was on hepatitis C and you have downloaded 100 reprints on this topic in your Documents folder. Your focus has now become more detailed, and you are now interested in reviewing the literature on outcomes associated with specific treatments of this disease. You might consider starting a new master folder (which you could call Hepatitis C Tx Outcomes Lit Review master) and begin to download reprints on this topic.

As you create and use these lit review master folders, you might want to truncate the names to something manageable, such as Hep C Outcomes master folder and the corresponding Hep C Outcomes Documents folder or Hep C Outcomes Paper Trail.

It is useful to always include a standard set of names in your folders so you can perform a quick and reliable search of your desktop for information. For example, searching for master folders could produce all of the master folders you have created for any literature review.

## HOW TO UPDATE A LITERATURE REVIEW EFFICIENTLY

If you review the literature on a topic once and never look at those source documents or return to that topic again, then you can skip this section. If, however, you need to evaluate new information or consider source documents added since the original review on the same subject, then you need a strategy for updating your review of the literature. One of the simplest ways to do this is to abstract the source documents you have added since the last review and bring the review matrix up to date.

A typical scenario for an experienced scientist is one in which an extensive review of the literature is prepared as part of a grant proposal, and then the Lit Review master folder, including the Documents folder and review matrix, is set aside during the period when the grant is reviewed. After the grant is awarded, then the research begins, with new references added to the reference library and new source documents stored in the Documents folder as they become available. Later, in preparing scientific papers about the results of the study, another thorough review of the literature is needed, probably with a more specific focus than in the grant proposal. The same lit review master folder can be used for all three purposes: generation of the initial literature review for the proposal, a documents folder for storing and adding reprints of source documents over time, and the preparation of the literature review for the manuscript describing the results of a completed study. Over the same period of time, from grant proposal to publication of research results, both the Documents folder and the Lit Review master folder have kept pace with the researcher.

In general, updating a review of the literature is more efficient, more thorough, and quicker if the materials are organized and updated as you go along. Materials such as a reference library, which might be available on a server that can be accessed by all members of a research team, and the Lit Review master folder, which might be stored in a central location for the same team, are invaluable resources that will help advance the research effort.

# Caroline's Quest: Using the Matrix Indexing System

In her review of the literature, Caroline was interested in exploring the possibility of a link between smoking by teenage girls and depression. As an initial step, she searched for a review article on depression. The process she used illustrates the Matrix Indexing System, from identifying the paper in the electronic bibliographic database to downloading the abstract with her reference management software to making a note that she had a copy of the article in the Documents folder in a lit review master folder.

Caroline began by logging onto PubMed on her computer and searched for a review article that she had identified earlier, one by Leon and colleagues.[2] She downloaded the reference and abstract onto her computer. Using EndNote, which was the reference management software Caroline had on her computer, she imported the reference and abstract into her Documents folder, which she had titled "Teenagers & Smoking References."

In the standard EndNote abstract form, she also wrote a note that she had a reprint of the entire article stored in the Documents folder within her Depression Lit Review master folder located in the master folder library.

Several days later, Caroline met with Professor Dickerson to discuss her progress. By this point she had a large file of reprints and was having trouble keeping track of them all. She asked, "What do you do when there are too many reprints? I can't create more and more documents folders."

"Well," he told her, "when that happens, you might think about organizing them by decade of publication." He pointed to the screen of his own computer, "For example, the 109 reprints I have on depression are located in three documents folders in the Depression Lit Review master folder, which I've separated chronologically by publication in 1980–1989, 1990–1994, and 1995–present. They are labeled Depression (1980–89) Documents, Depression (1990–94) Documents, and Depression (1995–present) Documents. Because they are indexed by year of publication, neither my students nor I have any problem finding a specific reprint."

Caroline made a note of Professor Dickerson's strategy for handling too many reprints and then returned to a discussion of her use of the Matrix Indexing System. "I guess this system could be used with any kind of literature review," she reflected, "whether or not it is of the scientific literature."

Professor Dickerson described how a colleague who was an author of a series of books on gardening used the Matrix Indexing System for keeping track of his notes, gardening catalogs, and reprints from popular magazines about gardening tips. "It really is a sensible way of organizing a lot of material," he agreed.

# REFERENCES

1. Turabian KL. *A Manual for Writers of Term Papers, Theses, and Dissertations.* 6th ed. Chicago, IL: University of Chicago Press; 1996.
2. Leon AC, Klerman GL, Wickramaratne P. Continuing female predominance in depressive illness. *Am J Public Health.* 1993;83:754–757.

# 9 Matrix Applications by Health Sciences Professionals

The purpose of this chapter is to describe examples of how the Matrix Method and the Matrix Indexing System can be used in some of the more advanced research and development activities in the health sciences. These examples are included in the following sections in the chapter:

- ⊙ What Are Matrix Applications?
- ⊙ How to Use Matrix Applications in a Research Project
- ⊙ How to Use Matrix Applications in a Meta-Analysis
- ⊙ How to Use Matrix Applications in Practice Guidelines
- ⊙ How to Use Matrix Applications in Evidence-Based Medicine
- ⊙ Caroline's Quest: Matrix Applications in a Nonscientific Setting

# WHAT ARE MATRIX APPLICATIONS?

A Matrix Application is the use of the concepts and procedures of the Matrix Method, the Matrix Indexing System, or both. The Matrix Method is a plan for gathering materials to be included in a review of the literature, systematically analyzing the information, writing a synthesis, and organizing and filing documents, notes, and other materials in one of four sections (paper trail folder, documents folder, review matrix folder, or synthesis folder) in a lit review master folder during and after completion of the review. The Matrix Indexing System is a set of procedures for bringing together and accessing information from three locations: (1) references obtained from electronic bibliographic databases, (2) a documents folder on your computer, and (3) copies of scientific papers and other materials stored in the Documents folder within your master folder.

## Advantages of Matrix Applications

Used either separately or together, the Matrix Method and the Matrix Indexing System offer an efficient strategy that can be used throughout the career of a health sciences professional in a variety of settings, including the following:

- Academia
- Research and evaluation consulting firms
- Clinical settings such as a private practice or managed care organization
- City, county, and state departments of health and public health
- Government and health policy organizations responsible for policy analysis or development of health legislation and regulations
- Research and development departments in private sector and health-related industries such as pharmaceutical or medical electronics companies
- Consumer health information organizations such as those that produce science magazines and newsletters, patient information brochures for managed care organizations or hospitals, and health and science sections of daily newspapers

Matrix applications can be used by an individual or by a group or team of people. For example, in setting up a matrix indexing system for use by a group, the Documents folder created with reference management software such as EndNote or RefWorks could be maintained on a server or office computer that is accessible to all members of a research or development team. Reprints of the research papers and other scientific articles filed chronologically in the Documents folder also could be maintained in a central location, and a system for adding new source documents and accessing them could be developed among members of the team.

When used together, the Matrix Method and the Matrix Indexing System offer a versatile and effective strategy for conducting a review of the literature and maintaining a library of reprints by an individual or group in a variety of settings. This is a cost- and time-efficient strategy for the busy health sciences professional. Examples of how this strategy can be used in the context of different kinds of activities are described in the remainder of this chapter.

The example used in "Caroline's Quest" at the end of this chapter departs from the traditional scientific setting and describes how matrix applications can be modified and used in preparing background information for a lay audience. Whether the author's intent is to communicate research findings to a group of scientists or to describe the latest breakthrough in medicine to readers of a daily newspaper, matrix applications can be used to organize the writer's reprints, notes, and thoughts.

## HOW TO USE MATRIX APPLICATIONS IN A RESEARCH PROJECT

A typical research project has several stages of development, from the conception of the idea to publication of the final results. These stages may vary depending on the researcher, the reason for doing the project, and the goals of the research. In an academic setting, research projects in the health sciences generally follow these three stages: (1) preparation of a proposal describing the hypothesis and methods for carrying out the study (sometimes this is a grant proposal, which is a request for funding of the study), (2) implementation of the project after approval or funding has been obtained, and (3) preparation of the written reports and papers to be submitted for publication in peer-reviewed journals.

The Matrix Method and Matrix Indexing System can be used to access, analyze, and manage references, reprints, and reviews of the literature at each of these three stages in the research process. Application of these tools also can have a cumulative advantage as the information and the files acquired at each stage build on those gathered at the previous stage.

For example, preparing a grant proposal is rarely a linear activity that progresses in lockstep from the generation of an idea, to reviewing of the literature, to planning the methodology, to writing the proposal. In reality, these activities occur more or less simultaneously. Although each of these tasks may dominate the researcher's time and attention at any point in time, there is often the need to recheck the literature while in the midst of planning the methodology or to rethink the research questions as plans for the proposed analysis are being finalized.

Most experienced researchers will have a working knowledge of the research literature as they think about ideas for a new study for months or even years. As these thoughts germinate, additional possibilities for studies may be suggested in publications or presentations at scientific meetings or in discussions with colleagues. Additional publications, such as newly published journal articles, can be stored in a documents folder within a lit review master folder and indexed in a documents folder on the scientist's computer.

When ideas for a research study begin to take shape, a more intensive effort may be mounted to review the literature systematically, especially on topics tangentially related to the research idea or to methodological approaches that might be applicable. At this point, a review matrix can be set up, the choice of column topics made, and the research literature abstracted.

Finally, when the grant proposal or other research document is written, the intensity will increase in tracking down specific references or locating studies in areas in which there appear to be gaps in the knowledge base. This is the point when a synthesis is written, based on the literature abstracted in the review matrix.

By developing and maintaining a matrix indexing system from the mulling-over period to its use in the preparation of a review matrix, researchers can accumulate the materials they need to abstract the literature and write a concise synthesis. Often there is a strict limitation on the number of pages in a grant proposal. The literature review, which is one small part of the proposal, has to be accurate, thorough, and concise. For example, most National Institutes of Health grant proposals have a 25-page limit, of which the literature review is a very small part. Therefore, previous knowledge about the topic has to be distilled and thoroughly accurate. The review matrix is a useful tool in this distillation process.

After the research project is funded, the researcher will continue to read the scientific literature and download new publications to the Documents folder, using reference management software such as RefWorks to maintain an up-to-date reprint file of the relevant studies. Later, when the project has progressed to the preparation of scientific papers or reports, the health scientist with an up-to-date documents folder in his or her lit review master folder is in a good position to update the review matrix of previously abstracted papers and write a synthesis for the papers.

# HOW TO USE MATRIX APPLICATIONS IN A META-ANALYSIS

A meta-analysis consists of the statistical evaluation of multiple research studies or clinical trials on a specific topic. Standardized procedures for conducting a meta-analysis are summarized in Chapter 3, and some historical background about the development of the meta-analytic technique is described in Chapter 1.

The procedures for a meta-analysis require that a study protocol be clearly specified. The first task is to describe the purpose, the methodology, and especially the criteria for selecting studies. Next the studies to be analyzed must be selected and reviewed. Finally, the statistical procedures for summarizing the results are applied to the set of studies included in the analysis.

The Matrix Method provides a structure for carrying out the first two stages of a meta-analysis. For example, the criteria for the kinds of studies to be gathered and a complete record of how the literature was searched can be documented in the Paper Trail folder located in the Lit Review master folder. After the studies for the meta-analysis are selected, they can be assembled and filed chronologically in the

Documents folder. Then the critical elements of purpose and research methodology can be abstracted in a review matrix. The information needed for the statistical analysis can also be included as column topics in the review matrix.

The advantage of using the Matrix Method becomes even more apparent if the meta-analysis is being done by two or more people. Often, a large number of scientific papers have to be reviewed before a final decision is made about which studies meet the criteria. This task could be assigned to two or more people who use a review matrix with the same set of column topics. Then the final selection of the studies to be included in the meta-analysis could be based on the information abstracted in their review matrices.

The primary emphasis in a meta-analysis is on the statistical summary of empirical studies and the interpretation of those results; however, these end points could be compromised by the ways in which the tasks of selecting and reviewing the basic materials—the studies to be analyzed—are carried out. The Matrix Method and the Matrix Indexing System provide an additional level of organization and efficiency in rigorously accomplishing those fundamental tasks for a meta-analysis.

Although this guide is tailored largely to graduate students for use in an academic setting, the Matrix Method and the Matrix Indexing System are applicable to research in other arenas as well. The following two sections outline the use of the matrix applications for developing clinical practice guidelines and for performing research for evidence-based medicine.

## HOW TO USE MATRIX APPLICATIONS IN PRACTICE GUIDELINES

Practice guidelines give healthcare providers such as physicians, nurses, and allied health professionals sound strategies for delivering the best possible health care based on the scientific literature. Although practice guidelines initially were created by nationally based teams of healthcare professionals under the sponsorship of organizations such as the Agency for Healthcare Research and Quality, recently such development has shifted to more local or regional groups made up of clinicians within managed care organizations, healthcare reimbursement companies, and even small practice groups.

The fundamental concept in developing a clinical practice guideline is to create a set of best practices for diagnosing, treating, managing, or preventing a clinical condition based on the scientific literature. Regardless of what practice guideline is being developed, a review of the literature is a necessary step, and matrix applications can be an integral part of this phase of the development of a practice guideline.

Consider, for example, a team of clinicians in an outpatient clinic consisting of a pediatric nurse practitioner, a pediatrician, and a telephone triage or intake nurse who work together to develop a practice guideline on otitis media (middle ear infection) in young children. After agreeing on the definition of the condition and the criteria for the guideline, they divide the task of reviewing the literature based on the process and the structure of the Matrix Method.

The intake nurse reviews the literature on symptoms of the condition. The pediatrician focuses on current research on treatment and clinical management, and the nurse practitioner concentrates on studies about prevention of otitis media at the individual and community levels. By coordinating their efforts through the use of a single lit review master folder, the task is accomplished in less time than it would take an individual. For example, they meet to agree on the criteria for the search, maintain a log of the strategies they used and the electronic databases and other sources they consulted, and generate an ongoing list of key words. This information is recorded in the Paper Trail folder within their Lit Review master folder, which is stored in a central location. The documents they gather, including reprints of studies, examples of guidelines from other groups, and papers from secondary and tertiary sources such as the Cochrane Library, are filed in the Documents folder. Later in the process, they make a joint decision about the column topics to be included in a review matrix.

In abstracting the documents in the review matrix, the strategy they choose is to have all three team members carefully read all of the documents, but have different members abstract a subset of the column topics. For example, the nurse practitioner abstracts all of the documents for column topics concerned with treatment and management, and the pediatrician abstracts the same set of articles on recognition of symptoms. Thus, by the time the guideline is ready to be written, all of the team members are thoroughly versed in the scientific literature.

In this example, the column topics might include methodological issues, but the focus is on the major subheadings of the guideline, such as symptom recognition, diagnosis, treatment, management, and prevention. The purpose of the guideline will dictate the choice of column topics for the review matrix.

The Matrix Indexing System would also be an asset in preparing a clinical guideline as the literature is being reviewed and then later in updating the guideline. For example, once a year, a member of the original team uses the same search strategy with the same electronic bibliographic database, such as MEDLINE, to identify new studies on the same topic. During the same period of time, team members or any of the other practitioners in the outpatient clinic add scientific papers or other materials to the Documents folder within the Otitis Media Lit Review master folder located on the server for the office. One person in the clinic is designated as the individual responsible for coordinating all lit review master folders on a variety of clinical topics of interest to the clinicians.

In summary, matrix applications will not accomplish all of the tasks needed to develop clinical practice guidelines, but they can provide an efficient process and a well-defined structure for accomplishing the task. Matrix applications can also be especially useful when a team of health professionals must coordinate their efforts to produce a single product in the form of a guideline for the care of patients with a specific condition.

## HOW TO USE MATRIX APPLICATIONS IN EVIDENCE-BASED MEDICINE

Evidence-based medicine is as much a philosophy about the importance of using current research findings as a basis for clinical decisions as it is a series of well-defined users' guides for understanding how to read and interpret the literature. Currently, there are 32 users' guides and more are expected in the future.[1-32] The Matrix Method and Matrix Indexing System are consistent with the principles of evidence-based medicine and can provide a structure and process for implementing this approach.

Consider, for example, a nurse practitioner in a diabetes clinic who wants to develop an outpatient program on diet and exercise for her older patients that would emphasize improvement in their quality of life. She begins by reading the users' guide published in the 1997 issue of *JAMA* on how to use articles about health-related quality of life.[17]

After she understands the principles of this type of research as described in that users' guide, she begins her search of the current literature. She also stores a copy of the users' guide in front of the Paper Trail folder within her Diabetes Lit Review master folder in order to have it handy.

Using the principles of the Matrix Method, she looks up the users' guide on MEDLINE and records the medical subject headings, some of which include quality of life, quality-adjusted life years, and patient care planning. She then searches MEDLINE for this type of article in combination with key words describing the condition such as diabetes, diet, and exercise. She also examines the list of references at the end of the users' guide on health-related quality of life in order to identify studies that might be related to her topic of interest.

Although her focus is on the quality of life of older people, she realizes that research in this area is relatively recent and might not have included people over 65 years old. For that reason, she does not limit her MEDLINE search by age of subjects. She keeps notes in the Paper Trail folder within her Lit Review master folder on the key words, procedures, and search strategies she used.

After reviewing references and abstracts of the studies online, she downloads the references from MEDLINE into a documents folder on her computer using EndNote. Next she uses MEDLINE to search for specific articles and downloads those that are most relevant to her topic. In deciding which column topics to use in setting up the review matrix, the nurse practitioner again consults the users' guide on health-related quality of life. She includes as column topics some of the issues raised in that article, such as whether the research studies she reviews measured aspects of patients' lives that the patients themselves considered important, and characteristics of the data collection instruments, especially the validity of the questionnaire. In general, the users' guide helps the nurse practitioner think about the kinds of issues that she needs to consider in her own review of the literature.

After abstracting the research studies in the review matrix, the nurse practitioner writes a brief synthesis of the literature as a basis for deciding which instrument to use in measuring health-related quality of life in her clinical practice. In the process of identifying research studies from MEDLINE, she creates a documents folder on health-related quality of life and uses a location label to note which references had a downloaded copy of the complete study in the Documents folder within her Quality of Life Lit Review master folder.

# Caroline's Quest:
# Matrix Applications in a Nonscientific Setting

One of the requirements of the master's degree program Caroline was enrolled in was a 3-month internship in the community. Caroline was interested in applying what she had learned in her public health courses to helping people in the community understand and use current research findings to improve their own health. She therefore chose to do her internship with a science writer for a local city newspaper. Caroline's first assignment was to do background research for a three-part series of articles to be published in the newspaper on how to prevent injuries to children in day care centers.

The newspaper's health reporter responsible for the final writing of the series of articles was Caroline's mentor for the internship. Together they developed an outline that Caroline would follow to gather information needed for writing the articles. The topics for the three articles were (1) a description of the kinds of injuries to children in day care settings and what their causes are, (2) how such injuries can be prevented, and (3) a checklist for parents to use as they determined whether a day care center was safe.

Caroline began by searching some of the major electronic bibliographic databases, including MEDLINE from 1985 to the present, Current Contents from 1994 to the present, and CINAHL from 1982 to the present. She found three research studies from these sources.[33–35] She downloaded each of these papers into her Documents folder.

Next, Caroline called the state health department and talked to the director of the office responsible for licensing day care centers about the reporting of day care injuries. She recorded her notes on a standard interview form, shown in Exhibit 9-1. Caroline also obtained a copy of the statistics for fatal and nonfatal injuries to day care children over the past five years. She made a pdf file copy of her notes and stored this pdf file in her Documents folder.

| Exhibit | |
|---|---|
| **9-1** | **Caroline's Interview Form** |

Date _____   Time _____

Person interviewed _____

Telephone _____   Fax _____

E-mail _____

Company/organization _____

Interview topic _____

Notes and quotes _____

_____

_____

Additional contacts or leads suggested _____

_____

Caroline's reporter-mentor looked over the information Caroline had collected and advised her to do some telephone interviews with experts in the field.

"How do I locate the experts?" Caroline asked. "Maybe I could try to call the authors of the research articles?" she looked inquisitively at the reporter.

Her mentor smiled, "Yes, but a quicker way to solve that problem would be to contact the people at ProfNet and find out whether there are any local experts with information that would be of interest to the our readers."

"What's ProfNet?" Caroline asked.

"It's an Internet service staffed by public relations experts at colleges and universities across the country that provides journalists and authors with leads on expert sources from more than 4,000 colleges, universities, think tanks, national laboratories, hospitals, nonprofit organizations, corporations, and public relations agencies. It was founded in 1992. Our newspaper has a subscription to this service. Look up their website; I'll send you the link. The ProfNet section you should access for this series of articles is Health/Medicine." The mentor sent her a link to ProfNet—http://profnet3.prnewswire.com/enter/index.jsp.

As a result of her inquiries on ProfNet, Caroline contacted professors at two nearby universities and a staff person at a nonprofit organization for prevention of childhood injuries. She recorded her notes from each interview on her standardized interview form.

During the first week of her internship, Caroline also searched other sites on the Internet, such as some of the leading newspapers, state and federal agencies responsible for regulation of day care centers, and local and statewide associations of licensed day care providers. From these sources, she identified parents, day care providers, and community leaders who were willing to be interviewed. She called several people from each of these categories.

Caroline used the Matrix Method to organize the information she collected for the newspaper assignment. First, she created a lit review master folder with the usual four folders: paper trail, documents, review matrix, and synthesis. In the Paper Trail folder, she documented her search activities and added a subsection on interviews where she kept a list of interviewees by date and other people they suggested that she contact. This list was actually a record of her use of the snowball technique applied to people, rather than references, as Professor Dickerson had taught her initially.

Caroline modified the standard approach of the Matrix Method to her needs in this nonscientific setting. First, she expanded the Documents folder within the Lit Review master folder by adding three subfolders: research studies, interviews, and statistics. After she had collected sufficient information, Caroline broadened the idea of column topics for the review matrix. She used the broad headings of the three-part series to develop three subtopics, consisting of research studies, interviews (further subdivided by parents, day care providers, regulators, experts, and other), and statistics. In constructing the review matrix, Caroline treated each type of information as a document, whether it was a research study, a set of notes on a standardized interview form, or a list of statistics. By using the review matrix in this way, she was better able to see what was missing and where she needed additional information. Caroline then wrote a brief three-page memo synthesizing the information from the review matrix— one page for each of the three intended articles.

While in the process of preparing the Lit Review master folder on day care injuries, Caroline also used the Matrix Indexing System to either download information from an electronic source, such as MEDLINE, or enter notes directly into a word processing document on her desktop computer. In addition to the standard EndNote templates for a journal article, book, or report, Caroline also had the option of using a template for a newspaper article, a personal communication (which she used to record each of the interviews), and a generic format, which she used to make a record of her statistical reports.

As they were going over the final materials in preparation for writing the three-part series, Caroline's reporter-mentor was surprised by the effort Caroline had gone to in organizing the background information. "This is a lot of work!" her mentor commented. "Usually I just keep a few notes on a yellow legal pad from which I write the article."

"I know it seems like extra effort," Caroline replied, "but actually, it's a lot easier to have it all in the same spot—in the Lit Review master folder—where I can just grab the whole set when I need it. Storing everything in a master folder, together with a downloaded copy of each article in the Documents folder, also helps me keep track of where things are for other writing assignments. I can't always remember where I put a downloaded copy of a study or the notes of an interview, but I can usually recall which assignment I was working on. Then all I have to do is go to the master folder on that assignment. It's called the Matrix Method."

Caroline's mentor commented, "Seems to me that the Matrix Method is useful in a lot of ways when it is necessary to summarize information. I think I'll try it myself."

"Oh, yes," Caroline said a bit smugly, "it's a very useful strategy. Even from the beginning, I knew that the Matrix Method was more than just a simple spreadsheet that's called a review matrix."

Caroline raised her eyebrows a bit like Professor Dickerson did when he began a lecture, "The Matrix Method is a system for how to access, integrate, and use information from a variety of sources in order to prepare a written synthesis of the scientific literature. I recommend it highly."

# REFERENCES

1. Guyatt GH, Rennie D. Users' guides to the medical literature. *JAMA*. 1993;270:2096–2097.

2. Oxman AD, Sackett DL, Guyatt GH. Users' guides to the medical literature: I: How to get started. *JAMA*. 1993;270:2093–2095.

3. Guyatt GH, Sackett DL, Cook DJ, for the Evidence-Based Medicine Working Group. Users' guides to the medical literature: II: How to use an article about therapy or prevention: A: Are the results of the study valid? *JAMA*. 1993; 270:2598–2601.

4. Guyatt GH, Sackett DL, Cook DJ, for the Evidence-Based Medicine Working Group. Users' guides to the medical literature: II: How to use an article about therapy or prevention: B: What were the results and will they help me in caring for my patients? *JAMA*. 1994;271:59–63.

5. Jaeschke R, Guyatt G, Sackett DL, for the Evidence-Based Medicine Working Group. Users' guides to the medical literature: III: How to use an article about a diagnostic test: A: Are the results of the study valid? *JAMA*. 1994;271:389–391.

6. Jaeschke R, Guyatt GH, Sackett DL, for the Evidence-Based Medicine Working Group. Users' guides to the medical literature: III: How to use an article about a diagnostic test: B: What are the results and will they help me in caring for my patients? *JAMA*. 1994;271:703–707.

7. Levine M, Walter S, Lee H, et al. Users' guides to the medical literature: IV: How to use an article about harm. *JAMA*. 1994;271:1615–1619.

8. Laupacis A, Wells G, Richardson WS, Tugwell P, for the Evidence-Based Medicine Working Group. Users' guides to the medical literature: V: How to use an article about prognosis. *JAMA*. 1994;272:234–237.

9. Oxman AD, Cook DJ, Guyatt GH, for the Evidence-Based Medicine Working Group. Users' guides to the medical literature: VI: How to use an overview. *JAMA*. 1994; 272:1367–1371.

10. Richardson WS, Detsky AS, for the Evidence-Based Medicine Working Group. Users' guides to the medical literature: VII: How to use a clinical decision analysis: A: Are the results of the study valid? *JAMA*. 1995;273:1292–1295.

11. Richardson WS, Detsky AS, for the Evidence-Based Medicine Working Group. Users' guides to the medical literature: VII: How to use a clinical decision analysis: B: What are the results and will they help me in caring for my patients? *JAMA*. 1995;273:1610–1613.

12. Hayward RS, Wilson MC, Tunis SR, Bass EB, Guyatt G, for the Evidence-Based Medicine Working Group. Users' guides to the medical literature: VIII: How to use clinical practice guidelines: A: Are the recommendations valid? *JAMA*. 1995;274:570–574.

13. Wilson MC, Hayward RS, Tunis SR, Bass EB, Guyatt G, for the Evidence-Based Medicine Working Group. Users' guides to the medical literature: VIII: How to use clinical practice guidelines: B: What are the recommendations and will they help you in caring for your patients? *JAMA*. 1995;274:1630–1632.

14. Guyatt GH, Sackett DL, Sinclair JC, et al. Users' guides to the medical literature: IX: A method for grading health care recommendations. *JAMA*. 1995;274:1800–1804.

15. Naylor CD, Guyatt GH, for the Evidence-Based Medicine Working Group. Users' guides to the medical literature: X: How to use an article reporting variations in the outcomes of health services. *JAMA*. 1996;275:554–558.

16. Naylor CD, Guyatt GH, for the Evidence-Based Medicine Working Group. Users' guides to the medical literature: XI: How to use an article about a clinical utilization review. *JAMA*. 1996;275:1435–1439.

17. Guyatt GH, Naylor CD, Juniper E, et al, for the Evidence-Based Medicine Working Group. Users' guides to the medical literature: XII: How to use articles about health-related quality of life. *JAMA*. 1997;277: 1232–1237.

18. Drummond MG, Richardson WS, O'Brien BJ, Levine M, Heyland D, for the Evidence-Based Medicine Working Group. Users' guides to the medical literature: XIII: How to use an article on economic analysis of clinical practice: A: Are the results of the study valid? *JAMA*. 1997;277:1552–1557.

19. O'Brien BJ, Heyland D, Richardson WS, Levine M, Drummond MF, for the Evidence-Based Medicine Working Group. Users' guides to the medical literature: XIII: How to use an article on economic analysis of clinical practice: B: What are the results and will they help me in caring for my patients? *JAMA*. 1997;277: 1802–1806.

20. Dans AL, Dans LF, Guyatt GH, Richardson S, for the Evidence-Based Medicine Working Group. Users' guides to the medical literature: XIV: How to decide on the applicability of clinical trial results to your patient. *JAMA*. 1998;279:545–549.

21. Richardson WS, Wilson MC, Guyatt GH, Cook DJ, Nishikawa J, for the Evidence-Based Medicine Working Group. Users' guides to the medical literature: XV: How to use an article about disease probability for differential diagnosis. *JAMA*. 1999;281:1214–1219.

22. Guyatt GH, Sinclair J, Cook DJ, Glasziou P, for the Evidence-Based Medicine Working Group and the Cochrane Applicability Methods Working Group. Users' guides to the medical literature: XVI: How to use a treatment recommendation. *JAMA*. 1999;281:1836–1843.

23. Barratt A, Irwig L, Glasziou P, et al., for the Evidence-Based Medicine Working Group. Users' guides to the medical literature: XVII: How to use guidelines and recommendations about screening. *JAMA*. 1999;281:2029–2034.

24. Randolph AG, Haynes RB, Wyatt JC, Cook DJ, Guyatt GH, for the Evidence-Based Medicine Working Group. Users' guides to the medical literature: XVIII: How to use an article evaluating the clinical impact of a computer-based clinical decision support system. *JAMA*. 1999;282:67–74.

25. Bucher HC, Guyatt GH, Cook DJ, Holbrook A, McAlister FA, for the Evidence-Based Medicine Working Group. Users' guides to the medical literature: XIX: Applying clinical trial results: A: How to use an article measuring the effect of an intervention on surrogate end points. *JAMA*. 1999;282:771–778.

26. McAlister FA, Laupacis A, Wells GA, Sackett DL, for the Evidence-Based Medicine Working Group. Users' guides to the medical literature: XIX: Applying clinical trial results: B: Guidelines for determining whether a drug is exerting (more than) a class effect. *JAMA*. 1999;282:1371–1377.

27. Hunt DL, Jaeschke R, McKibbon KA, Evidence-Based Medicine Working Group. Users' guides to the medical literature: XXI: Using electronic health information resources in evidence-based practice. *JAMA*. 2000;283:1875–1879.

28. McAlister FA, Straus SE, Guyatt GH, Haynes RB, Evidence-Based Medicine Working Group. Users' guides to the medical literature: XX: Integrating research evidence with the care of the individual patient. *JAMA*. 2000;283:2829–2836.

29. McGinn TG, Guyatt GH, Wyer PC, et al., for the Evidence-Based Medicine Working Group. Users' guides to the medical literature: XXII: How to use articles about clinical decision rules. *JAMA*. 2000;284:79–84.

30. Giacomini MK, Cook DJ, Evidence-Based Medicine Working Group. Users' guides to the medical literature: XXIII: Qualitative research in health care: B: What are the results and how do they help me care for my patients? *JAMA*. 2000;284:478–482.

31. Richardson WS, Wilson MC, Williams JW Jr, Moyer VA, Naylor CD, for the Evidence-Based Medicine Working Group. Users' guides to the medical literature: XXIV: How to use an article on the clinical manifestations of disease. *JAMA*. 2000;284:869–875.

32. Guyatt GH, Haynes RB, Jaeschke RZ, et al. Users' guides to the medical literature: XXV: Evidence-based medicine: Principles for applying the users' guides to patient care. *JAMA*. 2000;284:1290–1296.

33. Strauman-Raymond K, Lie L, Kempf-Berkseth J. Creating a safe environment for children in day care. *J School Health*. 1993;63:254–257.

34. Bernardo LM. Parent-reported injury-associated behaviors and life events among injured, ill, and well preschool children. *J Pediatr Nursing*. 1996;11:100–110.

35. Williams AF, Wells JAK, Ferguson SA. Development and evaluation of programs to increase proper child restraint use. *J Safety Res*. 1997;28:197–202.

Appendix

# A

# Useful Resources for Literature Reviews

## PURPOSE

This appendix consists of lists of sources and resources that may be useful in searching for information as you review the literature. Resources on
the Internet as well as the more standard print
sources are provided. Website addresses were accurate at the time that this book went to press, but
these addresses can change; the author and publisher assume no responsibility for their continued accuracy. If the address is not accurate when
you use it, then try using the key words of the organization in a general search for the correct
address.

# USEFUL REFERENCES AND LISTS FOR THE HEALTH SCIENCES PROFESSIONAL

## Clinical Practice Guidelines

*Electronic Source*

> Institute of Medicine of the National Academies (http://www.iom.edu)

*Print Sources*

> American Medical Association. *Clinical Practice Guidelines Directory: 1999–2000 Ed.* Chicago, IL: American Medical Association; 2000.
>
> Green E, Katz J, eds. *Clinical Practice Guidelines for the Adult Patient.* St. Louis, MO: Mosby; 1994.
>
> Lechtenberg R, Schutta HS, eds. *Neurology Practice Guidelines.* New York, NY: M. Dekker; 1998.
>
> National Comprehensive Cancer Network. *Oncology practice guidelines. Oncology.* 1996;10(11 Suppl), pp. 3–317.
>
> United States: U.S. Preventive Services Task Force. *Guide to Clinical Preventive Services: Recommendations of the U.S. Preventive Services Task Force.* 3rd ed. Washington, DC: Agency for Healthcare Research and Quality; 2005. Also available at http://www.ahrq.gov/clinic/uspstfix.htm.

## Periodicals about Clinical Practice Guidelines

> Centers for Disease Control and Prevention. *Morbidity and Mortality Weekly Report (MMWR)*: http://www.cdc.gov/mmwr.
>
> Joint Commission on Accreditation of Healthcare Organizations. *Abstracts of Clinical Care Guidelines. 1989–present.* Monthly abstracts of guidelines.
>
> U.S. Department of Health and Human Services, Agency for Health Care Policy and Research. *Guide to Clinical Preventive Services: Report of the U.S. Preventive Services Task Force, to United States: U.S. Preventive Services Task Force. Guide to clinical preventive services:*

Recommendations of the U.S. Preventive Services Task Force. 3rd ed. Washington, DC: Agency for Healthcare Research and Quality; 2005. Also available at http://www.ahrq.gov/clinic/uspstfix.htm.

## Additional References about Clinical Guidelines

Cook DJ, Greengold NL, Ellrodt AG, Weingarten SR. The relations between systematic reviews and practice guidelines. *Ann Intern Med.* 1997;127:210–216.

Field MJ, Lohr KN, eds. *Guidelines for Clinical Practice: From Development to Use. Committee on Clinical Practice Guidelines, Division of Health Care Services, Institute of Medicine.* Washington, DC: National Academy Press; 1992. Also available at Guidelines for Clinical Practice: From Development to Use.

Lohr KN. Guidelines for clinical practice: What they are and why they count. *J Law Med Ethics.* 1995;23:49–56.

Saver, BG. Whose guideline is it, anyway? [editorial]. *Arch Fam Med.* 1996;5:532–534.

## Evidence-Based Medicine: List of Users' Guides by Year of Publication

### 1993 Users' Guides

Guyatt GH, Rennie D. Users' guides to the medical literature [editorial]. *JAMA.* 1993;270:2096–2097.

Guyatt GH, Sackett DL, Cook DJ, for the Evidence-Based Medicine Working Group. Users' guides to the medical literature: II: How to use an article about therapy or prevention: A: Are the results of the study valid? *JAMA.* 1993;270:2598–2601.

Oxman AD, Sackett DL, Guyatt GH. Users' guides to the medical literature: I: How to get started. *JAMA.* 1993;270:2093–2095.

### 1994 Users' Guides

Guyatt GH, Sackett DL, Cook DJ, for the Evidence-Based Medicine Working Group. Users' guides to the medical literature: II: How to use an article about therapy or prevention: B: What were the results and will they help me in caring for my patients? *JAMA.* 1994;271:59–63.

Jaeschke R, Guyatt G, Sackett DL, for the Evidence-Based Medicine Working Group. Users' guides to the medical literature: III: How to use an article about a diagnostic test: A: Are the results of the study valid? *JAMA.* 1994;271:389–391.

Jaeschke R, Guyatt GH, Sackett DL, for the Evidence-Based Medicine Working Group. Users' guides to the medical literature: III: How to use an article about a diagnostic test: B: What are the results and will they help me in caring for my patients? *JAMA.* 1994;271:703–707.

Laupacis A, Wells G, Richardson WS, Tugwell P, for the Evidence-Based Medicine Working Group. Users' guides to the medical literature: V: How to use an article about prognosis. *JAMA.* 1994; 272:234–237.

Levine M, Walter S, Lee H, et al. Users' guides to the medical literature: IV: How to use an article about harm. *JAMA.* 1994;271: 1615–1619.

Oxman AD, Cook DJ, Guyatt GH, for the Evidence-Based Medicine Working Group. Users' guides to the medical literature: VI: How to use an overview. *JAMA.* 1994;272:1367–1371.

## *1995 Users' Guides*

Guyatt GH, Sackett DL, Sinclair JC, et al. Users' guides to the medical literature: IX: A method for grading health care recommendations. *JAMA.* 1995;274:1800–1804.

Hayward RS, Wilson MC, Tunis SR, Bass EB, Guyatt G, for the Evidence-Based Medicine Working Group. Users' guides to the medical literature: VIII: How to use clinical practice guidelines: A: Are the recommendations valid? *JAMA.* 1995;274:570–574.

Richardson WS, Detsky AS, for the Evidence-Based Medicine Working Group. Users' guides to the medical literature: VII: How to use a clinical decision analysis: A: Are the results of the study valid? *JAMA.* 1995;273:1292–1295.

Richardson WS, Detsky AS, for the Evidence-Based Medicine Working Group. Users' guides to the medical literature: VII: How to use a clinical decision analysis: B: What are the results and will they help me in caring for my patients? *JAMA.* 1995;273:1610–1613.

Wilson MC, Hayward RS, Tunis SR, Bass EB, Guyatt G, for the Evidence-Based Medicine Working Group. Users' guides to the medical literature: VIII: How to use clinical practice guidelines: B: What are the recommendations and will they help you in caring for your patients? *JAMA.* 1995;274:1630–1632.

## 1996 Users' Guides

Naylor CD, Guyatt GH, for the Evidence-Based Medicine Working Group. Users' guides to the medical literature: X: How to use an article reporting variations in the outcomes of health services. *JAMA.* 1996;275:554–558.

Naylor CD, Guyatt GH, for the Evidence-Based Medicine Working Group. Users' guides to the medical literature: XI: How to use an article about a clinical utilization review. *JAMA.* 1996;275: 1435–1439.

## 1997 Users' Guides

Drummond MG, Richardson WS, O'Brien BJ, Levine M, Heyland D, for the Evidence-Based Medicine Working Group. Users' guides to the medical literature: XIII: How to use an article on economic analysis of clinical practice: A: Are the results of the study valid? *JAMA.* 1997;277:1552–1557.

Guyatt GH, Naylor CD, Juniper E, for the Evidence-Based Medicine Working Group. Users' guides to the medical literature: XII: How to use articles about health-related quality of life. *JAMA.* 1997;277: 1232–1237.

O'Brien BJ, Heyland D, Richardson WS, Levine M, Drummond MF, for the Evidence-Based Medicine Working Group. Users' guides to the medical literature: XIII: How to use an article on economic analysis of clinical practice: B: What are the results and will they help me in caring for my patients? *JAMA.* 1997;277:1802–1806.

## 1998 Users' Guide

Dans AL, Dans LF, Guyatt GH, Richardson S, for the Evidence-Based Medicine Working Group. Users' guides to the medical literature: XIV: How to decide on the applicability of clinical trial results to your patient. *JAMA.* 1998;279:545–549.

## 1999 Users' Guides

Barratt A, Irwig L, Glasziou P, et al., for the Evidence-Based Medicine Working Group. Users' guides to the medical literature: XVII: How to use guidelines and recommendations about screening. *JAMA.* 1999;281:2029–2034.

Bucher HC, Guyatt GH, Cook DJ, Holbrook A, McAlister FA, for the Evidence-Based Medicine Working Group. Users' guides to the medical literature: XIX: Applying clinical trial results: A: How to use an article measuring the effect of an intervention on surrogate end points. *JAMA.* 1999;282:771–778.

Guyatt GH, Sinclair J, Cook DJ, Glasziou P, for the Evidence-Based Medicine Working Group and the Cochrane Applicability Methods Working Group. Users' guides to the medical literature: XVI: How to use a treatment recommendation. *JAMA.* 1999;281: 1836–1843.

McAlister FA, Laupacis A, Wells GA, Sackett DL, for the Evidence-Based Medicine Working Group. Users' guides to the medical literature: XIX: Applying clinical trial results: B: Guidelines for determining whether a drug is exerting (more than) a class effect. *JAMA.* 1999; 282:1371–1377.

Randolph AG, Haynes RB, Wyatt JC, Cook DJ, Guyatt GH, for the Evidence-Based Medicine Working Group. Users' guides to the medical literature: XVIII: How to use an article evaluating the clinical impact of a computer-based clinical decision support system. *JAMA.* 1999;282:67–74.

Richardson WS, Wilson MC, Guyatt GH, Cook DJ, Nishikawa J, for the Evidence-Based Medicine Working Group. Users' guides to the medical literature: XV: How to use an article about disease probability for differential diagnosis. *JAMA.* 1999;281:1214–1219.

## 2000 Users' Guides

Giacomini MK, Cook DJ, for the Evidence-Based Medicine Working Group. Users' guides to the medical literature: XXIII: Qualitative research in health care: A: Are the results of the study valid? *JAMA.* 2000;284:357–362.

Guyatt GH, Haynes RB, Jaeschke RZ, Cook DJ, Green L, Naylor CD, Wilson MC, Richardson WS, for the Evidence-Based Medicine Working Group. Users' guides to the medical literature: XXV:

Evidence-based medicine: principles for applying the users' guides to patient care. *JAMA*. 2000;284:1290–1296.

Hunt DL, Jaeschke R, McKibbon KA, for the Evidence-Based Medicine Working Group. Users' guides to the medical literature: XXI: Using electronic health information resources in evidence-based practice. *JAMA*. 2000;283:1875–1879.

McAlister FA, Straus SE, Guyatt GH, Haynes RB, for the Evidence-Based Medicine Working Group. Users' guides to the medical literature: XX: Integrating research evidence with the care of the individual patient. *JAMA*. 2000;283:2829–2836.

McGinn TG, Guyatt GH, Wyer PC, Naylor CD, Stiell IG, Richardson WS, for the Evidence-Based Medicine Working Group. Users' guides to the medical literature: XXII: How to use articles about clinical decision rules. *JAMA*. 2000;284:79–84.

Richardson WS, Wilson MC, Williams JW Jr, Moyer VA, Naylor CD, for the Evidence-Based Medicine Working Group. Users' guides to the medical literature: XXIV: How to use an article on the clinical manifestations of disease. *JAMA*. 2000;284:869–875.

## Users' Guides Published after 2000

For an updated list of users' guides published after 2000, consult the following book:

Guyatt G, Rennie D, Meade MO, Cook DJ. *Users' Guides to the Medical Literature: A Manual for Evidence-Based Clinical Practice*. 2nd ed. New York, NY: McGraw-Hill Companies/American Medical Association; 2008.

## Cochrane Reviews

A list of reviews is available at the Cochrane Collaboration website: http://www.cochrane.org.

## List of Annual Reviews by Category

Reviews of scientific information are published annually by Annual Reviews, which is a nonprofit scientific publisher. Current information about reviews can be found at the following website: http://www.annualreviews.org. Currently, there are 40 annual reviews in the following three categories, plus special publications on different topics. For an up-to-date list of all Annual Reviews publications, go to the following URL: http://www.annualreviews.org/catalog/index.aspx.

## Biomedical Sciences Publications

*Annual Review of Analytical Chemistry**
*Annual Review of Biochemistry*
*Annual Review of Biomedical Engineering*
*Annual Review of Biophysics and Biomolecular Structure**
*Annual Review of Cell and Developmental Biology*
*Annual Review of Chemical and Biomolecular Engineering**
*Annual Review of Clinical Psychology*
*Annual Review of Ecology, Evolution, and Systematics*
*Annual Review of Entomology*
*Annual Review of Food Science and Technology*
*Annual Review of Genetics*
*Annual Review of Genomics and Human Genetics*
*Annual Review of Immunology*
*Annual Review of Marine Science**
*Annual Review of Medicine*
*Annual Review of Microbiology*
*Annual Review of Neuroscience*
*Annual Review of Nutrition*
*Annual Review of Pathology: Mechanisms of Disease*
*Annual Review of Pharmacology and Toxicology*
*Annual Review of Physiology*
*Annual Review of Phytopathology*
*Annual Review of Plant Biology*
*Annual Review of Psychology**
*Annual Review of Public Health**

## Physical Sciences Publications

*Annual Review of Analytical Chemistry**
*Annual Review of Astronomy and Astrophysics*
*Annual Review of Biomedical Engineering*
*Annual Review of Biophysics and Biomolecular Structure**
*Annual Review of Chemical and Biomolecular Engineering**

*Annual Review of Condensed Matter Physics*
*Annual Review of Earth and Planetary Sciences*
*Annual Review of Environment and Resources* (Formerly *Energy and the Environment*)*
*Annual Review of Fluid Mechanics*
*Annual Review of Marine Science**
*Annual Review of Materials Research*
*Annual Review of Nuclear and Particle Science*
*Annual Review of Physical Chemistry*

## Social Sciences Publications

*Annual Review of Anthropology*
*Annual Review of Clinical Psychology**
*Annual Review of Environment and Resources**
*Annual Review of Law and Social Science*
*Annual Review of Political Science*
*Annual Review of Psychology**
*Annual Review of Public Health**
*Annual Review of Sociology*

## Economics

*Annual Review of Economics*
*Annual Review of Financial Economics*
*Annual Review of Resource Economics*

*Some of the series belong to more than one category.

## USEFUL RESOURCES

Boorkman JA, Huber JT, Roper FW. *Introduction to Reference Sources in the Health Sciences*. 4th ed. New York, NY: Neal-Schuman Publishers; 2004.

Bopp RE, Smith LC. *Reference and Information Services: An Introduction*. 2nd ed. Englewood, CO: Libraries, Unlimited; 1995.

Kuhlthau CC. *Seeking Meaning: A Process Approach to Library and Information Services*. Norwood, NJ: Ablex Publishing; 1993.

Kuhlthau CC. *Teaching the Library Research Process*. 2nd ed. Metuchen, NJ: The Scarecrow Press; 1994.

Lamm, K. *10,000 Ideas for Term Papers, Projects, Reports & Speeches*. New York, NY: Macmillan; 1995.

## USEFUL WEBSITES OF SCIENTIFIC ORGANIZATIONS, DIRECTORIES, PRINTED JOURNALS, AND ONLINE JOURNALS

American Anthropological Association (http://www.aaanet.org). Home page of the American Anthropological Association.

American Association for the Advancement of Science (http://www.aaas.org). Home page of the American Association for the Advancement of Science (AAAS). Includes links and information to many science fields.

American Chemical Society (http://www.chemistry.org). Home page of the American Chemical Society, with a membership of more than 151,000 chemists and chemical engineers.

American Institute of Biological Sciences (http://www.aibs.org). Home page of the American Institute of Biological Sciences, with links to BioScience Magazine.

*American Journal of Clinical Nutrition* (http://www.ajcn.org). Home page of the *American Journal of Clinical Nutrition*, which is a peer-reviewed journal that publishes basic and clinical studies relevant to human nutrition.

American Psychological Society (http://www.psychologicalscience.org). Home page of the American Psychological Society.

American Society for Biochemistry and Molecular Biology (http://www.asbmb.org). Home page of the American Society for Biochemistry and Molecular Biology.

American Society of Human Genetics (http://www.ashg.org). Home page of the American Society of Human Genetics.

American Sociological Association (http://www.asanet.org). Home page of the American Sociological Association.

BankIt: GenBank Submissions by WWW (http://www.ncbi.nlm.nih.gov/BankIt). Site for submitting genetic sequences and information on protein coding regions, mRNA features, and structural

RNA features to the GenBank library. Site is currently under revision.

CABI (http://www.cabi.org). Emphasis on agriculture, forestry, human health, and the management of natural resources, with particular attention to the needs of developing countries.

Center for the Advancement of Health (http://www.healthfinder. gov/orgs/hr2729.htm). The mission statement is "… The fundamental aim of the Center is to translate into policy and practice the growing body of evidence that can lead to improving and maintaining the health of individuals and the public."

Directory of Printed Periodicals (http://www.publist.com). A free online service that gives access to more than 150,000 printed periodicals throughout the world. Also provided is information about how to contact publishers, obtain rights and permissions, and receive documents. Initiated on the Web in June 1998. This website was being revised at the time this book was printed.

Federation of American Societies for Experimental Biology (http://www.faseb.org). Home page of the Federation of American Societies for Experimental Biology.

International Sociological Association (http://www.isa-sociology.org). Home page of the International Sociological Association.

*Journal of Biological Chemistry* (http://www.jbc.org). Online version of the *Journal of Biological Chemistry.*

*Journal of Cell Biology* (http://www.jcb.org). Online version of the *Journal of Cell Biology.*

*Journal of Clinical Investigation* (http://www.jci.org). Online version of the *Journal of Clinical Investigation.*

*Journal of Experimental Medicine* (http://www.jem.org). Online version of the *Journal of Experimental Medicine.*

*Journal of Nutrition* (http://nutrition.org). Published by the American Society for Nutritional Sciences. Online version of the *Journal of Nutrition,* which publishes papers based on original research in humans and other animal species.

*Journal Watch* (http://www.jwatch.org/). *Journal Watch* began in 1987 in both an online and newsletter format, reviewing the general medical literature for busy clinicians.

Lymphocyte Homing Images (http://www.geocities.com/Cape Canaveral/Hangar/1962). The site shows images from lymphocyte homing research.

National Academy of Sciences (http://www.nas.edu/). Home page of the National Academy of Sciences.

National Center for Biotechnology Information (http://www.ncbi.nlm.nih.gov/). A searchable molecular biology subset of MEDLINE with more than 1.5 million citations.

*Science Magazine* (http://www.sciencemag.org). Home page of *Science Magazine* Online with full text of print edition and science news section.

ScienceCareers.org (http://sciencecareers.sciencemag.org). A site for helping new scientists find jobs and keep up with new developments in their careers.

Society for Neuroscience (http://www.sfn.org). Dedicated to understanding the brain, spinal cord, and peripheral nervous system.

SocioSite (http://www.sociosite.net). Site for sociologists with a European and worldwide horizon.

Thomson Scientific (http://science.thomsonreuters.com/index.html). Publisher of Current Contents and the Science Citation Index.

The Vaccine Place (http://vaccines.com). This site collects, organizes, and presents news and annotated links about vaccines for parents, patients, practitioners, researchers, and students. Material is updated continuously.

# B Structure of Computer Folders for the Matrix Method

This appendix provides you with step-by-step instructions for creating a structure of computer folders for the Matrix Method on your desktop. These instructions assume you want to set up an arrangement of computer folders and blank documents before you begin your review of the literature. At the end of this appendix, there are answers to frequently asked questions about some of these suggestions and a complete example of an infrastructure of folders and files.

# FOLDER STRUCTURE

## Master Folder

Create a master folder for each literature review you conduct. Include a one-word descriptor as the topic for each master folder. For example, if you are planning to conduct two separate literature reviews, one on the public health effects of flooding and the other on prevention of malaria, then you would have two master folders:

>Lit Review master folder—Flooding
>Lit Review master folder—Malaria

See Chapter 7 for additional details about the creation and use of master folders.

## Subfolders

In each master folder, include four subfolders, corresponding to the four major parts of the Matrix Method. Include the topic label after each. Here are two examples:

>Lit Review master folder—Flooding
>>Paper Trail folder—Flooding
>>Documents folder—Flooding
>>Review Matrix folder—Flooding
>>Synthesis folder—Flooding

>Lit Review master folder—Malaria
>>Paper Trail folder—Malaria
>>Documents folder—Malaria
>>Review Matrix folder—Malaria
>>Synthesis folder—Malaria

See Chapter 7 for additional details.

## Specific Folders or Documents

Within each of the folders, you will place additional documents or folders as you progress through the Matrix Method. Here are some suggestions for your initial setup for each of the folders.

## Paper Trail Folder

In the Paper Trail folder, create five word processing documents. These will be blank at first, but you will use them to store notes as you progress through your review of the literature. Since you are creating them all at once, it will be easy to add the topic name when saving each document.

> Paper Trail folder—topic
>> Key Words—topic
>> Key Sources—topic
>> Electronic Bibliographic Databases—topic
>> URLs—topic
>> Notes—topic

See Chapter 3 for additional details about the Paper Trail folder.

## Documents Folder

This is the folder where you will keep a pdf file or other downloaded copy of each paper you select for your review. I find it easiest to begin by creating additional folders in the Documents folder by decade of publication in which to store these papers. Thus, if the literature review extends from 1980 to 2004, then I might create three folders for papers published between 1980 and 89, between 1990 and 99, from 2000 to 09, and from 2010 to the present. Of course I label each folder as follows:

> Documents folder—topic
>> Documents—topic, 1980–89
>> Documents—topic, 1990–99
>> Documents—topic, 2000–09
>> Documents—topic, 2010–present

Other ways of storing these documents could be used. For example, if you were organizing the papers in a literature review of the public health effects of flooding, you might organize by age of victim (infants, children, adults, elderly) or by global area in which the flooding occurred (North America, Central America, South America, Western Europe, Other Areas). Your goal in creating these folders is to have a well-understood location for storing the large number of studies you are likely to download in your review of the literature.

See Chapter 4 for more details about the Documents folder.

## Review Matrix Folder

In conducting a literature review, you will create a review matrix. Initially, when this was a paper-and-pencil system, there was only one matrix, which couldn't be easily reorganized. If your matrix has been created electronically, especially with a spreadsheet program such as Microsoft Excel, then you have the ability to sort that file in many different ways. My suggestions are these:

- **Review Matrix: Original**. Create an original review matrix (in an Excel file) based on the chronological order of publications. Store this in a separate folder in the review matrix folder, labeled "Original Review Matrix—topic."
- **Review Matrix: Methods Sort**. Make a copy of this original file and sort the rows (the papers you abstracted) by any of the columns. For example, you might sort your matrix by methodological rigor. If you labeled each paper by type of methodological design (experimental, quasiexperimental, preexperimental, or observational), then you could go to the methods column and sort by those key words. Such an arrangmentment might result in an alphabetical order, which might not be what you want. For example, the sort may result in an alphabetical arrangement, where experimental studies might be followed by observational studies, then pre-experimental and then quasi-experimental. That is not a logical order for the methodological designs, so you may have to manually rearrange the group of studies corresponding to the type of methodological design until the matrix is in the order you want. This arrangement would enable you to write a synthesis of the papers with the most rigorous designs. Alternatively, you might sort the original matrix by age group of subjects (children, adults, elderly). Of course, you have to have included those keywords in the appropriate column in order to use them as sorting keys.
- **Review Matrix: Another Sort**. Store each review matrix you sort in a separate folder in this review matrix folder. Organizing the literature in different ways is part of the thinking process in writing a synthesis of the literature. Before sorting the review matrix, record the criteria you used to create the sorting instructions

and store that information at the bottom of the first sheet of the sorted matrix.

See Chapter 5 for more details about the review matrix.

## Synthesis Folder

The Synthesis folder is the folder where you will keep a copy of all versions of your synthesis. At the end of each working session or day, save your draft of the synthesis and date stamp it. Here is an example of some the drafts of the synthesis documents you would store in this folder:

Synthesis folder—topic
    Synthesis—topic—7-20-09 original
    Synthesis—topic—7-23-09
    Synthesis—topic—7-24-09
    Synthesis—topic—7-28-09 final

Note that these are word processing documents, not folders. You could use date stamped folders if you wanted to simply store each copy of your synthesis manuscript in that folder, but that may require too much time or effort. Either way, maintain a copy of the synthesis each time you make major edits and keep those copies in this folder. It might also be helpful to tag the original and the final versions of your manuscript.

See Chapter 6 for more information about writing a synthesis.

# FREQUENTLY ASKED QUESTIONS

1. Why repeat the topic on the folders or files?

    Documents can get lost or misassigned to other folders, sometimes with just an accidental flick of the wrist. By routinely adding a topic tag to your folders or files, you can always use a find command to locate errant files.

2. Why should I keep different drafts of the synthesis? Why not just continually modify the original version and keep that version?

    The first draft of the synthesis can often be a brain dump or a stream of consciousness narrative of the review. Generally, I use a no-holds-barred approach in writing this draft—with no page limits and usually very little editing. Sometimes there are creative insights in the original draft that I may not use when I edit the second or later drafts.

In general, keep your early drafts. Don't edit over them because you may edit out some of the details you wish you had later. By saving the original and each of the major rewrites, you may preserve information you wish you had in later drafts.

3. How can I easily identify these master folders?

Most word processing systems have a feature that allows the user to color code a file or document. I find it useful to assign the same color to all the master folders and this allows me to easily find them on my desktop.

4. Why would I want to assemble the review matrix folders from different literature reviews?

If you have two or more lit review master folders, you can compare the content of the same folders or documents across these different literature reviews. For example, on your desktop, you might have completed four literature reviews on different but related topics. You might decide to compare the review matrices across those topics. Because you have used the same title for the first three words for those documents, you could use the find command to call up review matrix original. You would also be able to restore these files to their original folders by noting the topic name.

Another possibility might be to compare different documents or folders across collaborators. For example, a team of five people working on a practice guideline in hand-washing techniques might want to compare the methods sort of their different review matrices prior to writing a synthesis together. By putting a copy of the complete lit review master folder by each team member on the same desktop (and tagging each file or folder with the person's identification), their review matrix—methods sort spreadsheets could be pulled together and compared. They could then be restored to their original folders when the task is done.

5. Why should I set up this elaborate structure of folders and files when all I have to do is write up the results of a review of the literature?

A review of the literature can be a multiday, multiweek process that requires time, thought, and organization. You need a plan for where to put your tools and your products as you progress toward completion of a synthesis. The reason to set up a structure of folders and files before starting your review is that if you don't, things get lost or merged or not saved at all as you progress through this complex task.

Creating a structure of folders and files is like building a set of shelves in a kitchen. When you cook a large meal, you need to know where the equipment is or can be stored, where the food is located, and where to put different dishes, such as the salad in the refrigerator and the hot dish in the oven to keep it warm before the meal is served. That infrastructure of shelves, appliances, and an understanding of the layout of the kitchen itself contribute to your getting the meal on the table. Enjoy!

# EXAMPLE OF FILE STRUCTURE FOR THE MATRIX METHOD

Lit Review master folder—Flooding
    Paper Trail folder—Flooding
        Key Words—Flooding
        Key Sources—Flooding
        Electronic Bibliographic Databases—Flooding
        URLs—Flooding
        Notes—Flooding
    Documents folder—Flooding
        Documents folder—Flooding, 1980–89
        Documents folder—Flooding, 1990–99
        Documents folder—Flooding, 2000–present
    Review Matrix folder—Flooding
        Review Matrix: original—Flooding
        Review Matrix: Methods Sort—Flooding
        Review Matrix: Age Group—Flooding
    Synthesis folder—flooding
        Synthesis—flooding—10/02/09
        Synthesis—flooding—10/08/09
        Synthesis—flooding—10/14/09

In general, the structure you are setting up consists of *word processing documents* in the Paper Trail folder and in the Synthesis folder, *spreadsheet documents* (or word processing documents using the table option) in the Review Matrix folder, and *folders* in the Documents folder. Although you can create a skeleton structure for the contents of the Paper Trail folder and the Documents folder before you start the actual literature review, bear in mind that what you include in the Review Matrix folder and the Synthesis folder will be created as your work progresses. It's good to set this infrastructure up in advance, but it is also helpful to know what else you need to do in the process of going through the Matrix Method.

# Index

Page numbers followed by *exhibit, table,* or *figure*
indicate exhibits, tables or figures, respectively.

# About the Author

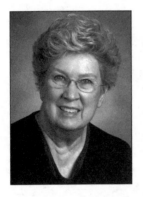

Judith Garrard, PhD, is a research psychologist with postgraduate training in epidemiology. She has been a professor at the University of Minnesota since 1971. She is the Senior Associate Dean for Academic Affairs and Research in the School of Public Health and professor in the Division of Health Policy and Management, School of Public Health.

Her teaching and research activities have been on a multidisciplinary basis throughout her career. For more than 35 years she taught graduate courses in research and program evaluation methods to students in public health, nursing, medicine, dentistry, veterinary medicine, and pharmacy, as well as those in education, psychology, and social work.

Dr. Garrard's research specialty is pharmacoepidemiology and patient outcomes, with a focus on prescription drug use by elderly people in the community, nursing homes, and assisted living facilities. She has authored or coauthored over 100 papers and reports, including peer-reviewed research papers on psychotropic drug use by elderly people. Over the past ten years, she has led a team of colleagues in pharmacy, neurology, and biostatistics in NIH-funded research on the use of antiepileptic drug use by nursing home residents. She has also been principal investigator or collaborator on numerous multidisciplinary research projects supported by NIH grants from the National Institute on Aging, National Institute for Neurological Diseases and Stroke, National Institute on Nursing, Agency for Health Care Policy Research, Health Care Financing Administration, Veterans Administration, and other granting agencies.

In 1990, Dr. Garrard received the Leonard M. Schuman Excellence in Teaching Award, and in 1991 a Career Research Award in social and behavioral geriatrics from the National Institute on Aging, NIH. In 1999, her book, *Health Sciences Literature Review Made Easy: The Matrix Method*, was published by Aspen Publications, Inc. The second and third editions were published by Jones and Bartlett Publishers in 2007 and 2010, respectively.